S0-CMS-513

# Procedure Checklists to Accompany

# FUNDAMENTALS OF NURSING: HUMAN HEALTH AND FUNCTION

*Ruth F. Craven and Constance J. Hirnle*

**Elissa Swisher Sauer,** RN, CS, MSN
**Chairman, Health Services Division**
**Director, Nursing Program**
**Reading Area Community College**
**Reading, Pennsylvania**

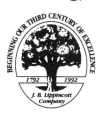

Acquisitions Editor: Donna L. Hilton, BSN, RN    Design Coordinator: Susan Hermansen
Coordinating Editorial Assistant: Susan Perry    Production Manager: Helen Ewan
Project Editor: Mary Rose Muccie                 Printer/Binder: Bawden Printing Inc.

Copyright © 1992, by J.B. Lippincott Company. All rights reserved. No part of this book may be used or reproduced in any manner whatsoever without written permission except for brief quotations embodied in critical articles and reviews. Printed in the United States of America. For information write J.B. Lippincott Company, 227 East Washington Square, Philadelphia, Pennsylvania 19106-3780.

ISBN: 0-397-54989-X

Any procedure or practice described in this book should be applied by the health-care practitioner under appropriate supervision in accordance with professional standards of care used with regard to the unique circumstances that apply in each practice situation. Care has been taken to confirm the accuracy of information presented and to describe generally accepted practices. However, the authors, editors, and publisher cannot accept any responsibility for errors or omissions or for any consequences from application of the information in this book and make no warranty, express or implied, with respect to the contents of the book.

Every effort has been made to ensure drug selections and dosages are in accordance with current recommendations and practice. Because of ongoing research, changes in government regulations and the constant flow of information on drug therapy, reactions and interactions, the reader is cautioned to check the package insert for each drug for indications, dosages, warnings and precautions, particularly if the drug is new or infrequently used.

# Procedure Checklists to Accompany

# FUNDAMENTALS OF NURSING: HUMAN HEALTH AND FUNCTION

## Preface

The Checklist Manual has been developed to provide faculty with a portable handbook to the procedures in the text: Fundamentals of Nursing: Human Health and Function. These checklists may be used during supervision of students' performance of procedures and may be reproduced for students to use as guidelines when practicing skills. They can also be modified to meet the needs of the situation, if desired.

The procedure steps in the checklists follow the steps of the procedures in the book with some minor modifications where needed for clarification. Where there are subsets of procedures, for example, measuring weight, a separate checklist is provided for each procedure. Thus, there are 110 checklists in this manual to correspond to the number of discrete procedures in the text. In these instances, in order to provide a complete procedure checklist, some of the introductory steps remain the same in each procedure but the subsequent steps vary. When this occurs, the procedure step number will deviate from the checklist step number even though the content is the same. In some other instances, the steps "Gather equipment", "Wash hands", "Document procedure and observations" has been added for continuity even though these may not appear in the procedure in the text.

It is hoped that this manual will be useful to you as you teach and supervise students in the nursing classroom laboratory or in a clinical experience.

© 1992 J.B. Lippincott Company, Fundamentals of Nursing: Human Health and Function

# Fundamentals of Nursing: Human Health and Function

## PROCEDURE CHECKLISTS

© 1992, J.B. Lippincott Company, Fundamentals of Nursing: Human Health and Function

## Procedure Checklists

# Procedure Checklists

© 1992, J.B. Lippincott Company, Fundamentals of Nursing: Human Health and Function

# PROCEDURE 18-1
## AUSCULTATING BREATH SOUNDS

|  |  | E | S | U |
|---|---|---|---|---|
| 1. | Wash hands. | [ ] | [ ] | [ ] |
| 2. | Assemble equipment. | [ ] | [ ] | [ ] |
| 3. | Assist patient to upright sitting position, lifting gown to expose chest. | [ ] | [ ] | [ ] |
| 4. | Warm diaphragm of stethoscope by holding between hands for a short time. | [ ] | [ ] | [ ] |
| 5. | Ask patient to breathe deeply, slowly, through mouth. | [ ] | [ ] | [ ] |
| 6. | Place diaphragm of stethoscope about 1 inch below the middle of the right clavicle, between the ribs. | [ ] | [ ] | [ ] |
| 7. | Listen for one full inspiration and exhalation on both sides of chest, noting normal and adventitious breath sounds. | [ ] | [ ] | [ ] |
| 8. | Move stethoscope downward about 1.5 to 2 inches along midclavicular line. Note sounds on both sides of chest. | [ ] | [ ] | [ ] |
| 9. | Move stethoscope downward to midclavicular line of fifth intercostal space, note sounds on both sides of chest. | [ ] | [ ] | [ ] |
| 10. | Instruct patient to lean forward, crossing arms in front. | [ ] | [ ] | [ ] |
| 11. | Auscultate area 2 inches below the shoulder and 2 inches to right of spine. Note sounds on both sides of chest. | [ ] | [ ] | [ ] |
| 12. | Move stethoscope downward 2 to 2.5 inches. Note sounds on both sides of chest. | [ ] | [ ] | [ ] |
| 13. | Move stethoscope downward 2 to 2.5 inches. Note sounds on both sides of chest. | [ ] | [ ] | [ ] |
| 14. | Move stethoscope downward to area just below scapula. Note sounds on both sides of chest. Listen laterally along rib cage. | [ ] | [ ] | [ ] |
| 15. | Replace patient's clothes and assist to comfortable position. | [ ] | [ ] | [ ] |
| 16. | Discuss findings with patient. | [ ] | [ ] | [ ] |
| 17. | Document assessment findings, being specific as to description of adventitious sounds and location. | [ ] | [ ] | [ ] |

E = Excels;  S = Satisfactory;  U = Unsatisfactory

COMMENTS:

[ ] Pass  [ ] Fail

Student's Signature_____  Date _____

Instructor's Signature_____  Date _____

© 1992 J.B. Lippincott Company, Fundamentals of Nursing: Human Health and Function

## PROCEDURE 18-2
## AUSCULTATING HEART SOUNDS

| | E | S | U |
|---|---|---|---|
| 1. Wash hands. | [ ] | [ ] | [ ] |
| 2. Assist patient to supine position, lifting gown to expose chest. | [ ] | [ ] | [ ] |
| 3. Warm diaphragm of stethoscope by holding between hands. | [ ] | [ ] | [ ] |
| 4. Listen in mitral area using diaphragm. Identify first and second heart sounds. Count heart rate, noting whether regular or irregular. If irregular, count for one minute. | [ ] | [ ] | [ ] |
| 5. Listen in aortic area using diaphragm. Concentrate on S1, then S2, systole, then diastole noting if splitting occurs. Listen for extra sounds. | [ ] | [ ] | [ ] |
| 6. Listen in pulmonic area using diaphragm. Concentrate on S1, S2, systole, diastole. Compare loudness of S2 in the aortic and pulmonic areas. | [ ] | [ ] | [ ] |
| 7. Listen in the tricuspid and mitral areas using diaphragm. | [ ] | [ ] | [ ] |
| 8. Assist to sitting position. Listen in aortic area, using bell of stethoscope. Concentrate on S1, S2, systole, and diastole. | [ ] | [ ] | [ ] |
| 9. Listen in pulmonic and tricuspid areas, using bell. | [ ] | [ ] | [ ] |
| 10. Listen in mitral area, using bell. Concentrate during diastole on S3 and S4. | [ ] | [ ] | [ ] |
| 11. Replace patient's clothes. Assist to comfortable position. | [ ] | [ ] | [ ] |
| 12. Record findings describing intensity, quality, and location of sounds. | [ ] | [ ] | [ ] |

E = Excels;  S = Satisfactory;  U = Unsatisfactory

COMMENTS:

[ ] Pass  [ ] Fail

Student's Signature_____ Date _____

Instructor's Signature_____ Date _____

© 1992 J.B. Lippincott Company, Fundamentals of Nursing: Human Health and Function

# PROCEDURE 18-3A
# MEASURING WEIGHT WITH STANDING SCALE

|  | E | S | U |
|---|---|---|---|
| 1. Wash hands. | [ ] | [ ] | [ ] |
| 2. Have patient void. | [ ] | [ ] | [ ] |
| 3. Remove slippers or shoes. Have patient wear same clothing for each weigh-in. | [ ] | [ ] | [ ] |
| 4. Place protection on scale. | [ ] | [ ] | [ ] |
| 5. Check that scale registers zero. Adjust if necessary. | [ ] | [ ] | [ ] |
| 6. Assist patient onto center of scale platform. Instruct not to lean or hold onto supports. | [ ] | [ ] | [ ] |
| 7. Read digital display or adjust counterweights to determine patient's weight. | [ ] | [ ] | [ ] |
| 8. Assist patient from scale. Dispose of protector sheet. | [ ] | [ ] | [ ] |
| 9. Record weight. | [ ] | [ ] | [ ] |

E = Excels;  S = Satisfactory;  U = Unsatisfactory

COMMENTS:

[ ] Pass  [ ] Fail

Student's Signature_____ Date _____

Instructor's Signature_____ Date _____

© 1992 J.B. Lippincott Company, Fundamentals of Nursing: Human Health and Function

4

# MEASURING WEIGHT WITH CHAIR SCALE

|  | | E | S | U |
|---|---|---|---|---|
| 1. | Wash hands. | [ ] | [ ] | [ ] |
| 2. | Have patient void. | [ ] | [ ] | [ ] |
| 3. | Remove slippers or shoes. Have patient wear same clothing for each weigh-in. | [ ] | [ ] | [ ] |
| 4. | Place protection on scale. | [ ] | [ ] | [ ] |
| 5. | Check that scale registers zero. Adjust if necessary. | [ ] | [ ] | [ ] |
| 6. | Place scale beside patient and lock wheels. | [ ] | [ ] | [ ] |
| 7. | Transfer patient onto chair. | [ ] | [ ] | [ ] |
| 8. | Read digital display or adjust counterweights to determine patient's weight. | [ ] | [ ] | [ ] |
| 9. | Transfer patient back to bed or wheelchair. Dispose of protector. | [ ] | [ ] | [ ] |
| 10. | Clean scale according to agency policy. | [ ] | [ ] | [ ] |
| 11. | Record weight. | [ ] | [ ] | [ ] |

E = Excels; S = Satisfactory; U = Unsatisfactory

COMMENTS:

[ ] Pass  [ ] Fail

Student's Signature_____ Date _____

Instructor's Signature_____ Date _____

© 1992 J.B. Lippincott Company, Fundamentals of Nursing: Human Health and Function

## PROCEDURE 18-3C
# MEASURING WEIGHT WITH BED SCALE

|  |  | E | S | U |
|---|---|---|---|---|
| 1. | Wash hands. | [ ] | [ ] | [ ] |
| 2. | Have patient void. | [ ] | [ ] | [ ] |
| 3. | Remove slippers or shoes.  Have patient wear same clothing for each weigh-in. | [ ] | [ ] | [ ] |
| 4. | Place protection on scale. | [ ] | [ ] | [ ] |
| 5. | Check that scale registers zero.  Adjust if necessary. | [ ] | [ ] | [ ] |
| 6. | Elevate patient's bed to level of stretcher scale. | [ ] | [ ] | [ ] |
| 7. | With one or two assistants, turn patient with back toward the scale. | [ ] | [ ] | [ ] |
| 8. | Roll scale toward bed, lock wheels in place, and lower stretcher onto bed. | [ ] | [ ] | [ ] |
| 9. | Attach stretcher arms to stretcher and gradually elevate stretcher about 2 inches above mattress surface. | [ ] | [ ] | [ ] |
| 10. | Inform patient before elevating.  Reassure that he will not fall but head may feel lower than body. | [ ] | [ ] | [ ] |
| 11. | Determine that stretcher is not touching any equipment.  Lift drains and tubing away from stretcher. | [ ] | [ ] | [ ] |
| 12. | Read digital display for patient's weight. | [ ] | [ ] | [ ] |
| 13. | Gradually lower stretcher to bed.  Remove stretcher arms and transfer patient off stretcher. Remove stretcher. | [ ] | [ ] | [ ] |
| 14. | Unlock bed scale wheels and move away from bed. | [ ] | [ ] | [ ] |
| 15. | Assist patient to comfortable position. | [ ] | [ ] | [ ] |
| 16. | Clean stretcher and scale according to agency policy. | [ ] | [ ] | [ ] |
| 17. | Record weight and note any extra linen or equipment weighed with the patient. | [ ] | [ ] | [ ] |

E = Excels;  S = Satisfactory;  U = Unsatisfactory

COMMENTS:

[ ] Pass  [ ] Fail

Student's Signature_____ Date _____

Instructor's Signature_____ Date _____

© 1992 J.B. Lippincott Company, Fundamentals of Nursing:  Human Health and Function

## PROCEDURE 18-4
## AUSCULTATING BOWEL SOUNDS

|  |  | E | S | U |
|---|---|---|---|---|
| 1. | Wash hands. | [ ] | [ ] | [ ] |
| 2. | Warm stethoscope. | [ ] | [ ] | [ ] |
| 3. | Ask patient when he or she last ate. | [ ] | [ ] | [ ] |
| 4. | Assist patient to a supine position with abdomen exposed. | [ ] | [ ] | [ ] |
| 5. | Place stethoscope diaphragm in each of the four quadrants of the abdomen. Listen for pitch, frequency, and duration of bowel sounds at each site. | [ ] | [ ] | [ ] |
| 6. | If bowel sounds not heard, listen for 3 to 5 minutes in all quadrants. | [ ] | [ ] | [ ] |
| 7. | Place stethoscope bell over the epigastrum. Listen for sounds associated with pulse rate. | [ ] | [ ] | [ ] |
| 8. | Cover patient and assist to comfortable position. | [ ] | [ ] | [ ] |
| 9. | Record findings. | [ ] | [ ] | [ ] |

E = Excels;  S = Satisfactory;  U = Unsatisfactory

COMMENTS:

[ ] Pass  [ ] Fail

Student's Signature_____  Date _____

Instructor's Signature_____  Date _____

© 1992 J.B. Lippincott Company, Fundamentals of Nursing:  Human Health and Function

# PROCEDURE 18-5
## ASSESSING THE NEUROLOGICAL SYSTEM

|  |  | E | S | U |
|---|---|---|---|---|
| 1. | Wash hands. | [ ] | [ ] | [ ] |
| 2. | Assemble equipment. | [ ] | [ ] | [ ] |
| 3. | Ask direct questions requiring a verbal response to assess level of consciousness. Note appropriateness of response and emotional state. | [ ] | [ ] | [ ] |
| 4. | Evaluate patient's speech patterns. | [ ] | [ ] | [ ] |
| 5. | Observe general appearance: hygiene, appropriateness of clothing to setting and weather. | [ ] | [ ] | [ ] |
| 6. | Ask direct questions of patient related to person, place and time if responses are inappropriate. | [ ] | [ ] | [ ] |
| 7. | Assess for communication or language problem. | [ ] | [ ] | [ ] |
| 8. | If patient doesn't or inappropriately responds to orientation questions, give simple commands (e.g."squeeze my fingers" or "wiggle your toes"). | [ ] | [ ] | [ ] |
| 9. | If there is no response to verbal commands, test response to painful stimuli by applying firm pressure on patient's sternum or finger nailbed with your thumb. | [ ] | [ ] | [ ] |
| 10. | Document level of consciousness objectively by stating specific patient responses to verbal or tactile stimulation. | [ ] | [ ] | [ ] |
| 11. | Assess function of cranial nerves. | [ ] | [ ] | [ ] |
|  | a. I (Olfactory) - Ask patient to identify different mild aromas like vanilla, coffee, chocolate, cloves. | [ ] | [ ] | [ ] |
|  | b. II (Optic) - Ask patient to read Snellen chart. | [ ] | [ ] | [ ] |
|  | c. III (Oculomotor) - Assess pupil reaction to penlight. | [ ] | [ ] | [ ] |
|  | d. III - Assess direction of gaze by holding finger 18 inches from patient's face. Ask patient to follow finger up and down and side to side. | [ ] | [ ] | [ ] |
|  | e. IV (Trochlear) - Assess direction of gaze while reading Snellen chart. | [ ] | [ ] | [ ] |
|  | f. V (Trigeminal) - Lightly touch cotton swab to lateral sclera of eye to elicit blink. | [ ] | [ ] | [ ] |
|  | g. V - Measure sensation of touch and pain on face with cotton wisp and pin. | [ ] | [ ] | [ ] |
|  | h. VI (Abducens) - Assess direction of gaze when testing cranial nerve III. | [ ] | [ ] | [ ] |
|  | i. VII (Facial) - Ask patient to smile, frown, raise eyebrows. | [ ] | [ ] | [ ] |
|  | j. VII - Ask patient to identify different tastes on tip and sides of tongue: sugar, salt, lemon juice. | [ ] | [ ] | [ ] |
|  | k. VIII (Auditory) - Assess ability to hear spoken word. | [ ] | [ ] | [ ] |
|  | l. IX (Glossopharyngeal) - Ask patient to identify different tastes on back of tongue (as in j.). | [ ] | [ ] | [ ] |

*(continued)*

© 1992 J.B. Lippincott Company, Fundamentals of Nursing: Human Health and Function

## 18-5: Assessing The Neurological System *(Continued)*

|  | E | S | U |
|---|---|---|---|
| m. IX - Place a tongue blade on posterior tongue while patient says "ah" to elicit gag response. | [ ] | [ ] | [ ] |
| n. IX - Ask patient to move tongue up and down, and side to side. | [ ] | [ ] | [ ] |
| o. X (Vagus) - Assess with cranial nerve IX by observing palate and pharynx move as patient says "ah". | [ ] | [ ] | [ ] |
| p. XI (Spinal Accessory) - Ask patient to turn head side to side and shrug shoulders against resistance from examiner's hands. | [ ] | [ ] | [ ] |
| q. XII (Hypoglossal) - Ask patient to stick out tongue to midline, then move it side to side. | [ ] | [ ] | [ ] |
| 12. Assess sensory pathways (patient's eyes are closed): | | | |
| a. Apply stimuli to skin in a random unpredictable order while comparing one side of body to the other. | [ ] | [ ] | [ ] |
| b. Note spinal cord segment affected if an area of altered sensation is detected. | [ ] | [ ] | [ ] |
| 13. Test pain sensation first by lightly touching pointed then blunt end of sterile pin to proximal and distal aspects of arms and legs. | [ ] | [ ] | [ ] |
| 14. Test temperature sensation by touching skin with vials of hot, then cold water. | [ ] | [ ] | [ ] |
| 15. Lightly stroke proximal and distal aspects of patient's arms and legs with a cotton ball. Ask patient to state when and where each stroke is felt. | [ ] | [ ] | [ ] |
| 16. Apply a vibrating tuning fork to the distal interphalangeal joint of fingers and great toe. Ask patient to what is felt and when it stops. | [ ] | [ ] | [ ] |
| 17. Grasp patient's finger. Move finger up and down asking patient to identify position. Repeat with toes. | [ ] | [ ] | [ ] |

## ACTIVITY-MOBILITY ASSESSMENT

|  | E | S | U |
|---|---|---|---|
| 18. Inspect arm and leg muscles for atrophy, tremors, fasiculations, or other abnormal movements. | [ ] | [ ] | [ ] |
| 19. Assess strength of specific muscle groups by having patient extend or flex individual joints against resistance provided by examiner's hands. Test biceps, triceps, wrist and leg muscles, and ankle. Evaluate for symmetry of same muscle groups. | [ ] | [ ] | [ ] |
| 20. Ask patient to close eyes and hold arms in front of body with palms up. Hold position for 30 seconds and observe for pronation of hands or drifting of arms. | [ ] | [ ] | [ ] |
| 21. Evaluate coordination and balance by: | | | |
| a. Have patient pat upper thigh by rapidly alternating palm and back of hand. | [ ] | [ ] | [ ] |

*(continued)*

© 1992 J.B. Lippincott Company, Fundamentals of Nursing: Human Health and Function

### 18-5:  Assessing The Neurological System *(Continued)*

|  | E | S | U |
|---|---|---|---|
| b. With dominant hand, have patient touch thumb to each finger on that hand as quickly as possible. | [ ] | [ ] | [ ] |
| c. Have patient use dominant forefinger to first touch your forefinger, then his or her nose repeatedly as fast as possible. | [ ] | [ ] | [ ] |
| d. Ask patient to stand with feet together, arms at sides.  Have patient maintain this position for 30 seconds with eyes open, then with eyes closed.  Assess for swaying.  (Romberg test) | [ ] | [ ] | [ ] |
| e. Ask patient to walk across room.  Observe gait for symmetry, rhythm, limping, shuffling, or other abnormalities. | [ ] | [ ] | [ ] |

22. Assess deep tendon reflexes (biceps, triceps, patellar, achilles) using the following technique:

|  | E | S | U |
|---|---|---|---|
| a. Compare symmetry of reflex on each side of body. | [ ] | [ ] | [ ] |
| b. Extremity to be tested should be completely relaxed and slightly extended. | [ ] | [ ] | [ ] |
| c. Reflex hammer should be held loosely and allowed to swing freely into an arc. | [ ] | [ ] | [ ] |
| d. Tap tendon briskly. | [ ] | [ ] | [ ] |
| e. Document reflexes by grading responses on a stickman figure: | [ ] | [ ] | [ ] |

    0 - no response
    1+ - diminished reflex
    2+ - normal
    3+ - brisker than normal
    4+ - hyperactive

|  | E | S | U |
|---|---|---|---|
| f. In newborn and infant, assess rooting, sucking, Moro, and tonic neck reflexes. | [ ] | [ ] | [ ] |

E = Excels;  S = Satisfactory;  U = Unsatisfactory

COMMENTS:

[ ] Pass  [ ] Fail

Student's Signature_____  Date_____

Instructor's Signature_____  Date_____

© 1992 J.B. Lippincott Company, Fundamentals of Nursing:  Human Health and Function

# PROCEDURE 19-1A
## ASSESSING BODY TEMPERATURE
### ORAL TEMPERATURE

|  |  | E | S | U |
|---|---|---|---|---|
| 1. | Wash hands. | [ ] | [ ] | [ ] |
| 2. | Explain procedure to patient. | [ ] | [ ] | [ ] |
| 3. | Put on disposable gloves if using a mercury thermometer. | [ ] | [ ] | [ ] |
| 4. | Remove thermometer from storage container and rinse with cold water. Dry with tissue. | [ ] | [ ] | [ ] |
| 5. | Hold thermometer at eye level. | [ ] | [ ] | [ ] |
| 6. | Check temperature reading on thermometer. If reading is not below 35° C., shake down by holding away from bulb between thumb and forefinger, and snap wrist sharply. Place plastic sheath on thermometer if using electronic thermometer. | [ ] | [ ] | [ ] |
| 7. | Place thermometer probe in patient's mouth in the posterior sublingual pocket. | [ ] | [ ] | [ ] |
| 8. | Ask patient to maintain thermometer position with lips closed. | [ ] | [ ] | [ ] |
| 9. | Leave in place 3 to 5 minutes with mercury thermometer, 10 to 20 seconds with electronic thermometer. Follow agency policy regarding recommended time interval. | [ ] | [ ] | [ ] |
| 10. | If using electronic thermometer, discard plastic sheath and read digital display. | [ ] | [ ] | [ ] |
| 11. | If using mercury thermometer, wipe off secretions with tissue. Hold thermometer at eye level and rotate it slowly until mercury column is visible. Note upper end of column as temperature reading. | [ ] | [ ] | [ ] |
| 12. | Wash mercury thermometer in soapy, tepid water. Rinse and replace in storage container. | [ ] | [ ] | [ ] |
| 13. | Remove gloves and wash hands. | [ ] | [ ] | [ ] |
| 14. | If using electronic thermometer, replace in battery charging unit. | [ ] | [ ] | [ ] |
| 15. | Document findings. | [ ] | [ ] | [ ] |

E = Excels;  S = Satisfactory;  U = Unsatisfactory

COMMENTS:


[ ] Pass  [ ] Fail

Student's Signature_____ Date _____


Instructor's Signature_____ Date _____

© 1992 J.B. Lippincott Company, Fundamentals of Nursing:  Human Health and Function

# PROCEDURE 19-1B
## ASSESSING BODY TEMPERATURE
### AXILLARY TEMPERATURE

|  | E | S | U |
|---|---|---|---|
| 1. Wash hands. | [ ] | [ ] | [ ] |
| 2. Explain procedure to patient. | [ ] | [ ] | [ ] |
| 3. Remove thermometer from storage container and rinse with cold water. Dry with tissue. | [ ] | [ ] | [ ] |
| 4. Hold thermometer at eye level. | [ ] | [ ] | [ ] |
| 5. Check temperature reading on thermometer. If reading is not below 35° C., shake down by holding away from bulb between thumb and forefinger, and snap wrist sharply. Place plastic sheath on thermometer if using electronic thermometer. | [ ] | [ ] | [ ] |
| 6. Close bedroom door or bed curtains. Assist patient to comfortable position, and expose axilla. | [ ] | [ ] | [ ] |
| 7. Insert thermometer into middle of axilla; fold patient's arm down and place across chest. | [ ] | [ ] | [ ] |
| 8. Hold in place 9 minutes in adults, 5 minutes in children. | [ ] | [ ] | [ ] |
| 9. If using electronic thermometer, discard plastic sheath and read digital display. | [ ] | [ ] | [ ] |
| 10. If using mercury thermometer, wipe off secretions with tissue. Hold thermometer at eye level and rotate it slowly until mercury column is visible. Note upper end of column as temperature reading. | [ ] | [ ] | [ ] |
| 11. Wash mercury thermometer in soapy, tepid water. Rinse and replace in storage container. | [ ] | [ ] | [ ] |
| 12. If using electronic thermometer, replace in battery charging unit. | [ ] | [ ] | [ ] |
| 13. Document findings. | [ ] | [ ] | [ ] |

E = Excels;  S = Satisfactory;  U = Unsatisfactory

COMMENTS:

[ ] Pass  [ ] Fail

Student's Signature_____ Date _____

Instructor's Signature_____ Date _____

© 1992 J.B. Lippincott Company, Fundamentals of Nursing: Human Health and Function

## PROCEDURE 19-1C
## ASSESSING BODY TEMPERATURE
### RECTAL TEMPERATURE

|  |  | E | S | U |
|---|---|---|---|---|
| 1. | Wash hands. | [ ] | [ ] | [ ] |
| 2. | Explain procedure to patient. | [ ] | [ ] | [ ] |
| 3. | Put on disposable gloves if using a mercury thermometer. | [ ] | [ ] | [ ] |
| 4. | Remove thermometer from storage container and rinse with cold water. Dry with tissue. | [ ] | [ ] | [ ] |
| 5. | Hold thermometer at eye level. | [ ] | [ ] | [ ] |
| 6. | Check temperature reading on thermometer. If reading is not below 35° C., shake down by holding away from bulb between thumb and forefinger, and snap wrist sharply. Place plastic sheath on thermometer if using electronic thermometer. | [ ] | [ ] | [ ] |
| 7. | Close bedroom door or bed curtains. Assist patient to Sim's position with upper leg flexed. Expose only anal area. | [ ] | [ ] | [ ] |
| 8. | Apply water soluble lubricant liberally to thermometer probe tip. | [ ] | [ ] | [ ] |
| 9. | Separate patient's buttocks with one hand to expose anus. | [ ] | [ ] | [ ] |
| 10. | Ask patient to take a deep, slow breath. Insert thermometer into anus in direction of umbilicus, for an infant 1/2", for an adult 1 1/2". Do not force. | [ ] | [ ] | [ ] |
| 11. | Hold in place 3 to 5 minutes according to agency policy. | [ ] | [ ] | [ ] |
| 12. | If using electronic thermometer, discard plastic sheath and read digital display. | [ ] | [ ] | [ ] |
| 13. | If using mercury thermometer, wipe off secretions with tissue. Hold thermometer at eye level and rotate it slowly until mercury column is visible. Note upper end of column as temperature reading. | [ ] | [ ] | [ ] |
| 14. | Wash mercury thermometer in soapy, tepid water. Rinse and replace in storage container. | [ ] | [ ] | [ ] |
| 15. | Remove gloves and wash hands. | [ ] | [ ] | [ ] |
| 16. | If using electronic thermometer, replace in battery charging unit. | [ ] | [ ] | [ ] |
| 17. | Document findings. | [ ] | [ ] | [ ] |

E = Excels;  S = Satisfactory;  U = Unsatisfactory

COMMENTS:

[ ] Pass  [ ] Fail

Student's Signature_____ Date _____

Instructor's Signature_____ Date _____

© 1992 J.B. Lippincott Company, Fundamentals of Nursing: Human Health and Function

## PROCEDURE 19-2A
## OBTAINING A PULSE
### RADIAL PULSE

|  | E | S | U |
|---|---|---|---|
| 1. Wash hands and explain procedure to patient. | [ ] | [ ] | [ ] |
| 2. Position patient comfortably with forearm across chest or at his/her side with wrist extended. | [ ] | [ ] | [ ] |
| 3. Place fingertips of your first three fingers along the groove at base of thumb, on patient's wrist. | [ ] | [ ] | [ ] |
| 4. Press against radial artery to obliterate pulse, then gradually release pressure until pulsations are felt. | [ ] | [ ] | [ ] |
| 5. Assess pulse for regularity and strength. | [ ] | [ ] | [ ] |
| 6. If pulse is not easily palpable, use Doppler: a. Apply conducting gel to end of probe or to radial site. | [ ] | [ ] | [ ] |
| b. Press "on" button and place probe against skin on pulse site. Reposition slightly using firm pressure until pulsating sound is heard. | [ ] | [ ] | [ ] |
| 7. If pulse is regular, count pulse for 15 seconds and multiply by four. If pulse is irregular, count for a full minute. | [ ] | [ ] | [ ] |
| 8. Document pulse on vital signs record. | [ ] | [ ] | [ ] |

E = Excels; S = Satisfactory; U = Unsatisfactory

COMMENTS:

[ ] Pass  [ ] Fail

Student's Signature_____ Date_____

Instructor's Signature_____ Date_____

© 1992 J.B. Lippincott Company, Fundamentals of Nursing: Human Health and Function

## PROCEDURE 19-2B
## OBTAINING A PULSE
### APICAL PULSE

|  | E | S | U |
|---|---|---|---|
| 1. Wash hands and explain procedure to patient. | [ ] | [ ] | [ ] |
| 2. Position patient in supine or sitting position with sternum and left chest exposed. | [ ] | [ ] | [ ] |
| 3. Warm diaphragm of stethoscope by holding in palm of hand for 5 to 10 seconds. | [ ] | [ ] | [ ] |
| 4. Insert the earpieces of stethoscope into your ears and place diaphragm over apex of patient's heart at fifth intercostal space, near midclavicular line. | [ ] | [ ] | [ ] |
| 5. Assess heartbeat for regularity and arrhythmias. | [ ] | [ ] | [ ] |
| 6. If rhythm is regular, count the heartbeat for 30 seconds and multiply by two. Count for a full minute if rhythm is irregular. | [ ] | [ ] | [ ] |
| 7. Replace patient's gown and assist in returning to a comfortable position. | [ ] | [ ] | [ ] |
| 8. Share results with patient. | [ ] | [ ] | [ ] |
| 9. Document pulse on vital signs record. | [ ] | [ ] | [ ] |

E = Excels;  S = Satisfactory;  U = Unsatisfactory

COMMENTS:

[ ] Pass  [ ] Fail

Student's Signature_____  Date_____

Instructor's Signature_____  Date _____

© 1992 J.B. Lippincott Company, Fundamentals of Nursing:  Human Health and Function

# PROCEDURE 19-3
# ASSESSING PULSE DEFICITS

|  |  | E | S | U |
|---|---|---|---|---|
| 1. | Wash hands. Explain procedure to patient. | [ ] | [ ] | [ ] |
| 2. | Introduce second examiner. Position patient comfortably. | [ ] | [ ] | [ ] |
| 3. | Remove clothing as necessary to select stethoscope placement site. Warm diaphragm of stethoscope by holding in hand. Place stethoscope over apex of heart. | [ ] | [ ] | [ ] |
| 4. | Second examiner places fingertips over radial artery pulse site. | [ ] | [ ] | [ ] |
| 5. | Place a watch where both examiners can clearly observe the second hand. Both examiners agree to start counting when the second hand reaches a predetermined number. | [ ] | [ ] | [ ] |
| 6. | Count the apical and radial rate for a full minute. | [ ] | [ ] | [ ] |
| 7. | Reposition patient and adjust clothing. | [ ] | [ ] | [ ] |
| 8. | Document apical and radial heart rates. | [ ] | [ ] | [ ] |

E = Excels;  S = Satisfactory;  U = Unsatisfactory

COMMENTS:

[ ] Pass  [ ] Fail

Student's Signature_____ Date_____

Instructor's Signature_____ Date _____

© 1992 J.B. Lippincott Company, Fundamentals of Nursing: Human Health and Function

## PROCEDURE 19-4
## ASSESSING RESPIRATIONS

|  | E | S | U |
|---|---|---|---|
| 1. After assessment of pulse, keep fingers resting on patient's wrist and observe or feel the rising and falling of chest with respiration. Do not explain procedure to patient. | [ ] | [ ] | [ ] |
| 2. When one complete cycle or inspiration and expiration has been observed, look at second hand of watch and count the number of complete cycles. If rate is regular in an adult, count 30 seconds and multiply by two. In children under 2 years of age or adults with irregular rate, count for a full minute. | [ ] | [ ] | [ ] |
| 3. Note depth and rhythm of respiratory cycle. | [ ] | [ ] | [ ] |
| 4. Discuss findings with patient, if applicable. | [ ] | [ ] | [ ] |
| 5. Document results. | [ ] | [ ] | [ ] |

E = Excels;  S = Satisfactory;  U = Unsatisfactory

COMMENTS:

[ ] Pass  [ ] Fail

Student's Signature_____ Date_____

Instructor's Signature_____ Date_____

© 1992 J.B. Lippincott Company, Fundamentals of Nursing: Human Health and Function

## PROCEDURE 19-5
## OBTAINING BLOOD PRESSURE

|  | E | S | U |
|---|---|---|---|
| 1. Wash hands. | [ ] | [ ] | [ ] |
| 2. Explain procedure to patient. | [ ] | [ ] | [ ] |
| 3. Assist patient to comfortable position with forearm supported at heart level and palm up. | [ ] | [ ] | [ ] |
| 4. Expose upper arm completely. | [ ] | [ ] | [ ] |
| 5. Wrap deflated cuff snugly around upper arm with center of bladder over brachial artery and lower border of cuff 2 cm. above antecubital space in an adult, nearer the antecubital space in an infant. | [ ] | [ ] | [ ] |
| 6. If using mercury manometer, the manometer is vertical and at eye level. | [ ] | [ ] | [ ] |
| 7. Palpate brachial or radial artery with fingertips. Close valve on pressure bulb and inflate cuff until pulse disappears. Inflate 30 mm. Hg. higher. Slowly release valve and note reading when pulse reappears. | [ ] | [ ] | [ ] |
| 8. Fully deflate cuff and wait 1 to 2 minutes. | [ ] | [ ] | [ ] |
| 9. Place stethoscope earpieces in ears. Repalpate the brachial artery and place stethoscope diaphragm or bell over site. | [ ] | [ ] | [ ] |
| 10. Close bulb valve and inflate cuff to 30 mm. Hg. above reading where brachial pulse disappeared. | [ ] | [ ] | [ ] |
| 11. Slowly release valve so pressure drops about 2 to 3 mm Hg. per second. | [ ] | [ ] | [ ] |
| 12. Identify manometer reading when first clear Korotkoff sound is heard. | [ ] | [ ] | [ ] |
| 13. Continue to deflate and note reading when sound muffles or dampens (fourth Korotkoff) and when it disappears (fifth Korotkoff). | [ ] | [ ] | [ ] |
| 14. Deflate cuff completely and remove from patient's arm. | [ ] | [ ] | [ ] |
| 15. Record blood pressure. Record systolic and diastolic in the form 130/80. If three readings are to be recorded, use the form 130/80/40. Abbreviate RA or LA to indicate right or left arm measurement. | [ ] | [ ] | [ ] |
| 16. Assist patient to comfortable position and discuss findings with patient, if appropriate. | [ ] | [ ] | [ ] |

E = Excels;  S = Satisfactory;  U = Unsatisfactory

COMMENTS:

[ ] Pass  [ ] Fail

Student's Signature_____ Date_____

Instructor's Signature_____ Date _____

© 1992 J.B. Lippincott Company, Fundamentals of Nursing: Human Health and Function

## PROCEDURE 19-6
# ASSESSING FOR ORTHOSTATIC HYPOTENSION

|  |  | E | S | U |
|---|---|---|---|---|
| 1. | Wash hands. Explain procedure to patient. | [ ] | [ ] | [ ] |
| 2. | Position patient supine with head of bed flat for 2 minutes. | [ ] | [ ] | [ ] |
| 3. | Check and record supine blood pressure and pulse. | [ ] | [ ] | [ ] |
| 4. | Assist patient to a sitting position with legs dangling over the edge of bed. Wait 2 minutes and check blood pressure and pulse rate. | [ ] | [ ] | [ ] |
| 5. | Assist patient to standing position. Wait 2 minutes and check blood pressure and pulse rate. Be alert to signs and symptoms of dizziness. | [ ] | [ ] | [ ] |
| 6. | Assist patient back to comfortable position. | [ ] | [ ] | [ ] |
| 7. | Record measurements and any symptoms that accompanied the postural change. | [ ] | [ ] | [ ] |
| 8. | Discuss the findings with patient, if appropriate. | [ ] | [ ] | [ ] |

E = Excels;  S = Satisfactory;  U = Unsatisfactory

COMMENTS:

[ ] Pass  [ ] Fail

Student's Signature_____ Date_____

Instructor's Signature_____ Date _____

© 1992 J.B. Lippincott Company, Fundamentals of Nursing: Human Health and Function

## PROCEDURE 20-1
# PREPARING THE PATIENT FOR DIAGNOSTIC PROCEDURES

|  |  | E | S | U |
|---|---|---|---|---|
| 1. | Identify the specific procedure or procedures to be performed. | [ ] | [ ] | [ ] |
| 2. | Obtain written consent for invasive procedures after the physician has explained the study to the patient. | [ ] | [ ] | [ ] |
| 3. | If more than one procedure is ordered, they should be scheduled in an order least traumatic to the patient and which will produce the most accurate results. | [ ] | [ ] | [ ] |
| 4. | Identify specific preparations needed to be performed before the procedure. | [ ] | [ ] | [ ] |
| 5. | Provide instruction to the patient and significant others regarding the procedure and rationale for any special preparations or dietary/fluid restrictions required by the study. | [ ] | [ ] | [ ] |
| 6. | Monitor dietary or fluid restrictions. Encourage eating or drinking well when not NPO. Schedule a rest day between procedures with dietary/fluid restrictions if possible. | [ ] | [ ] | [ ] |
| 7. | Continue to provide psychological support to the patient as needed. | [ ] | [ ] | [ ] |
| 8. | When patient who routinely takes special medications is NPO, obtain physician orders regarding administration of medications prior to the procedure. | [ ] | [ ] | [ ] |
| 9. | Immediately before the procedure: | | | |
| | a. Have patient urinate unless contraindicated by the study. | [ ] | [ ] | [ ] |
| | b. Reidentify any patient allergies. | [ ] | [ ] | [ ] |
| | c. Remove hairpins, contact lenses, jewelry, nail polish if required by the procedure. | [ ] | [ ] | [ ] |
| | d. Administer and document premedication if ordered. | [ ] | [ ] | [ ] |
| | e. If transported with intravenous line, assess that IV is patent and remaining volume is sufficient. | [ ] | [ ] | [ ] |
| | f. Supervise transfer from bed to wheelchair or gurney. If transported by gurney, side rails or safety belt is fastened. | [ ] | [ ] | [ ] |
| | g. Provide blanket. | [ ] | [ ] | [ ] |
| 10. | Accompany patient during transport if required by patient's physical or emotional status. | [ ] | [ ] | [ ] |

E = Excels;  S = Satisfactory;  U = Unsatisfactory

COMMENTS:

[ ] Pass  [ ] Fail

Student's Signature_____ Date_____

Instructor's Signature_____ Date _____

© 1992 J.B. Lippincott Company, Fundamentals of Nursing: Human Health and Function

## PROCEDURE 20-2
## MEASURING BLOOD GLUCOSE BY SKIN PUNCTURE

|  |  | E | S | U |
|---|---|---|---|---|
| 1. | Wash hands. | [ ] | [ ] | [ ] |
| 2. | Have patient wash hands with soap and warm water. | [ ] | [ ] | [ ] |
| 3. | Position patient at rest in comfortable position. | [ ] | [ ] | [ ] |
| 4. | Remove reagent strip from container and handle according to manufacturer's instructions. | [ ] | [ ] | [ ] |
| 5. | Place reagent strip with test pad up on dry surface. | [ ] | [ ] | [ ] |
| 6. | Choose the finger to be punctured, massage gently, and hold in dependent position. | [ ] | [ ] | [ ] |
| 7. | Wipe puncture site with alcohol. Allow to dry completely. | [ ] | [ ] | [ ] |
| 8. | Don gloves. | [ ] | [ ] | [ ] |
| 9. | Remove cover of lancet or autolet. Place autolet against side of finger and push release button. If lancet is used, it is held perpendicular to side of finger and pierces site quickly. | [ ] | [ ] | [ ] |
| 10. | Wipe initial drop of blood with cotton ball. | [ ] | [ ] | [ ] |
| 11. | Squeeze puncture gently or massage skin toward site to obtain large drop of blood. Hold reagent strip next to drop of blood and allow blood to cover the test pad completely. Do not smear blood. | [ ] | [ ] | [ ] |
| 12. | Start timing (usually 60 seconds) using glucose meter, or a watch if meter is not available. | [ ] | [ ] | [ ] |
| 13. | Following manufacturer's instruction, wipe blood from test pad with cotton ball after specified period of time. | [ ] | [ ] | [ ] |
| 14. | Place reagent strip into glucose meter. After recommended time period, read results. If glucose meter is not available, compare color of test pad with color strip on side of reagent strip container. | [ ] | [ ] | [ ] |
| 15. | Turn off glucose meter. Dispose of used equipment in appropriate manner. | [ ] | [ ] | [ ] |

E = Excels;  S = Satisfactory;  U = Unsatisfactory

COMMENTS:

[ ] Pass  [ ] Fail

Student's Signature_____  Date_____

Instructor's Signature_____  Date _____

© 1992 J.B. Lippincott Company, Fundamentals of Nursing: Human Health and Function

## PROCEDURE 22-1
## HANDWASHING

|  | E | S | U |
|---|---|---|---|
| 1. Remove all rings except a plain wedding band. Push watch 4 to 5 inches above wrist. | [ ] | [ ] | [ ] |
| 2. File nails short. Refrain from wearing nail polish or fake fingernails. | [ ] | [ ] | [ ] |
| 3. Turn on water and adjust temperature to warm. Do not splash water or lean against sink. | [ ] | [ ] | [ ] |
| 4. Hold hands lower than elbows and thoroughly wet hands and lower arms under running water. | [ ] | [ ] | [ ] |
| 5. Apply soap. If bar soap is used, rinse bar before lathering and rinse bar again before returning it to dish. | [ ] | [ ] | [ ] |
| 6. Rub palms, wrists, and back of hands firmly with circular movements. Interlace fingers and thumbs, moving hands back and forth. Continue using plenty of lather and friction for 15 to 20 seconds on each hand. | [ ] | [ ] | [ ] |
| 7. Clean under fingernails using fingernails of other hand and additional soap. Use orange-wood stick if available. | [ ] | [ ] | [ ] |
| 8. Rinse hands and wrists thoroughly with hands held lower than forearms. | [ ] | [ ] | [ ] |
| 9. Dry hands and arms thoroughly with paper towel, wiping from fingertips toward forearm. Discard towel in proper receptacle. | [ ] | [ ] | [ ] |
| 10. Turn off water using clean, dry paper towel on faucets. | [ ] | [ ] | [ ] |

E = Excels;  S = Satisfactory;  U = Unsatisfactory

COMMENTS:

[ ] Pass  [ ] Fail

Student's Signature_____ Date_____

Instructor's Signature_____ Date_____

© 1992 J.B. Lippincott Company, Fundamentals of Nursing: Human Health and Function

## PROCEDURE 22-2
# DONNING AND REMOVING A MASK AND GOWN

|  | E | S | U |
|---|---|---|---|

**DONNING MASK**

| | | E | S | U |
|---|---|---|---|---|
| 1. | Wash hands. | [ ] | [ ] | [ ] |
| 2. | If required, position mask over mouth and nose. Bend nose bar over bridge of nose. Secure strings or elastic. | [ ] | [ ] | [ ] |

**DONNING CLEAN GOWN**

| | | E | S | U |
|---|---|---|---|---|
| 1. | Grasp gown by collar allowing it to unfold. | [ ] | [ ] | [ ] |
| 2. | Place arms through sleeve and pull gown over shoulders. | [ ] | [ ] | [ ] |
| 3. | Fasten neck ties. Overlap gown at back and fasten waist ties. | [ ] | [ ] | [ ] |

**REMOVING CONTAMINATED GOWN**

| | | E | S | U |
|---|---|---|---|---|
| 1. | Untie waist ties and let hang freely. | [ ] | [ ] | [ ] |
| 2. | Wash hands. | [ ] | [ ] | [ ] |
| 3. | Untie neck ties and let gown fall forward off shoulders. | [ ] | [ ] | [ ] |
| 4. | Slide arms out of gown working from inside. | [ ] | [ ] | [ ] |
| 5. | Holding gown away from your body, fold contaminated side of gown toward the inside. | [ ] | [ ] | [ ] |
| 6. | Discard in appropriate receptacle. | [ ] | [ ] | [ ] |
| 7. | Remove and discard mask. | [ ] | [ ] | [ ] |
| 8. | Wash hands. | [ ] | [ ] | [ ] |

E = Excels;  S = Satisfactory;  U = Unsatisfactory

COMMENTS:

[ ] Pass  [ ] Fail

Student's Signature_____  Date_____

Instructor's Signature_____  Date _____

© 1992 J.B. Lippincott Company, Fundamentals of Nursing:  Human Health and Function

## PROCEDURE 22-3
## PRACTICING STRICT ISOLATION TECHNIQUE

|  | E | S | U |
|---|---|---|---|

**ENTERING A STRICT ISOLATION ROOM**

1. Wash hands.    [ ] [ ] [ ]
2. If clock is not available in room to use when taking pulse, remove watch and seal in plastic bag.    [ ] [ ] [ ]
3. Don mask, gown, gloves in hallway or anteroom. Pull cuff of gloves up over gown sleeves.    [ ] [ ] [ ]
4. Carry supplies into patient unit. Close door.    [ ] [ ] [ ]
5. Provide nursing care as necessary.    [ ] [ ] [ ]

**EXITING A STRICT ISOLATION ROOM**

6. Place contaminated linen into cloth or water dissolvable plastic bag, and close bag. Carry to doorway where second, nongloved health-care worker holds a large bag with cuff folded down over hands. Place first bag into second bag, being careful not to touch outside of second bag. Ungowned worker immediately closes bag and labels as isolation linen.    [ ] [ ] [ ]
7. Remove contaminated, disposable, or recyclable supplies from room using double-bagging technique.    [ ] [ ] [ ]
8. Untie waist ties of gown. Remove gloves and discard in patient's room. Wash hands. Untie neck ties.    [ ] [ ] [ ]
9. Remove gown by folding toward inside without touching the outside surfaces. Discard in room. Remove mask, and discard in room.    [ ] [ ] [ ]
10. Use clean, dry paper towel to open inside door handle. Leave room and close door from outside with bare hands.    [ ] [ ] [ ]
11. Wash hands.    [ ] [ ] [ ]

E = Excels;  S = Satisfactory;  U = Unsatisfactory

COMMENTS:

[ ] Pass  [ ] Fail

Student's Signature_____ Date_____

Instructor's Signature_____ Date_____

© 1992 J.B. Lippincott Company, Fundamentals of Nursing: Human Health and Function

## PROCEDURE 22-4
## APPLYING AND REMOVING STERILE GLOVES

| | E | S | U |
|---|---|---|---|
| **APPLYING GLOVES** | | | |
| 1. Wash hands. | [ ] | [ ] | [ ] |
| 2. Remove outside wrapper by peeling apart sides. | [ ] | [ ] | [ ] |
| 3. Lay inner package on clean, flat surface above waist level. Open wrapper from the outside keeping gloves on inside surface. | [ ] | [ ] | [ ] |
| 4. Grasp inside edge of right cuff with thumb and first two fingers of left hand. Holding hands above waist, insert right hand into glove. Adjust fingers inside glove after both gloves are on. | [ ] | [ ] | [ ] |
| 5. Slip gloved hand underneath second gloved cuff still in package, and pull over left hand. | [ ] | [ ] | [ ] |
| 6. Keeping hands above waist, adjust glove fit, touching only sterile areas. | [ ] | [ ] | [ ] |
| **REMOVING GLOVES** | | | |
| 7. With right hand, grasp outer surface of left glove just below thumb. Peel off without touching exposed wrist. | [ ] | [ ] | [ ] |
| 8. Place ungloved hand under thumbside of second cuff and peel off toward fingers, holding first glove inside second glove. Discard into appropriate receptacle. | [ ] | [ ] | [ ] |
| 9. Wash hands. | [ ] | [ ] | [ ] |

E = Excels; S = Satisfactory; U = Unsatisfactory

COMMENTS:

[ ] Pass [ ] Fail

Student's Signature______________________________ Date______________

Instructor's Signature______________________________ Date ______________

© 1992 J.B. Lippincott Company, Fundamentals of Nursing: Human Health and Function

## PROCEDURE 24-1
## ADMINISTERING ORAL MEDICATIONS

|  |  | E | S | U |
|---|---|---|---|---|
| 1. | Wash hands. | [ ] | [ ] | [ ] |
| 2. | Arrange medications kardex or cards next to medication cart or cabinet, medication trays and cups. | [ ] | [ ] | [ ] |
| 3. | Prepare medications for only one patient at a time. | [ ] | [ ] | [ ] |
| 4. | Remove ordered medication from cart or shelf. Compare label on medication with medication kardex or card. If there is a discrepancy, recheck the patient's chart and physician's orders. | [ ] | [ ] | [ ] |
| 5. | Calculate correct drug dosage if necessary. | [ ] | [ ] | [ ] |
| 6. | Prepare medications: |  |  |  |
|  | a. Unit dosage: Place packaged medication directly into medicine cup or lay on tray without unwrapping. | [ ] | [ ] | [ ] |
|  | b. Medications from multidose bottle: Pour tablets or capsules into container lid and transfer into medicine cup. Extra Tablets are returned to bottle without being touched. | [ ] | [ ] | [ ] |
|  | c. If patient cannot swallow tablets, crush in mortar with pestle until smooth. Mix in small amount of custard or applesauce if patient is permitted these foods. | [ ] | [ ] | [ ] |
|  | d. Liquid medications: Remove cap and place on container top upside down to prevent contamination. Hold bottle so label is against palm of hand. | [ ] | [ ] | [ ] |
|  | e. Hold medication cup at eye level and fill until bottom of meniscus is at desired dosage. Discard excess poured liquid from cup into sink not back into bottle. | [ ] | [ ] | [ ] |
|  | f. Oral narcotic: Compare previous drug count on narcotic record with current supply. Place drug in medication cup and record information on narcotic record. | [ ] | [ ] | [ ] |
| 7. | Compare prepared medication with medication kardex (or card) and container label. | [ ] | [ ] | [ ] |
| 8. | Reread label and place medication container or unused drug back on cart or shelf. | [ ] | [ ] | [ ] |
| 9. | Take medication directly to patient's room. Do not leave unattended. | [ ] | [ ] | [ ] |
| 10. | Ask patient to state his or her name and compare name on medication card or record with name on patient's identification band. | [ ] | [ ] | [ ] |
| 11. | Complete any preadministration assessment required by the specific medication. | [ ] | [ ] | [ ] |
| 12. | Explain purpose of medication to patient. | [ ] | [ ] | [ ] |
| 13. | Assist patient to sitting position. | [ ] | [ ] | [ ] |

*(continued)*

© 1992 J.B. Lippincott Company, Fundamentals of Nursing: Human Health and Function

26

## 24-1: Administering Oral Medications *(Continued)*

|  | E | S | U |
|---|---|---|---|
| 14. If using unit dose medications: Read label, unwrap medication, and place in cup. Give medication cup and glass of water or juice to patient. | [ ] | [ ] | [ ] |
| 15. If patient is unable to hold medication cup, place pill cup to lips and introduce medication into mouth. | [ ] | [ ] | [ ] |
| 16. Stay with patient until all medications are swallowed, checking inside mouth if necessary. | [ ] | [ ] | [ ] |
| 17. Dispose of soiled supplies and wash hands. | [ ] | [ ] | [ ] |
| 18. Record time medication was administered and any pre-administration assessment data which were collected. | [ ] | [ ] | [ ] |

E = Excels;  S = Satisfactory;  U = Unsatisfactory

COMMENTS:

[ ] Pass  [ ] Fail

Student's Signature_____ Date_____

Instructor's Signature_____ Date _____

© 1992 J.B. Lippincott Company, Fundamentals of Nursing:  Human Health and Function

## PROCEDURE 24-2A
## DRAWING UP TWO MEDICATIONS IN A SYRINGE

|  |  | E | S | U |
|---|---|---|---|---|
| 1. | Wash hands. | [ ] | [ ] | [ ] |
| 2. | Cleanse tops of both vials with antiseptic. | [ ] | [ ] | [ ] |
| 3. | With syringe, aspirate volume of air equal to medication dose from first medication (Vial A). | [ ] | [ ] | [ ] |
| 4. | Inject air into Vial A, being careful that needle does not touch solution. | [ ] | [ ] | [ ] |
| 5. | Remove syringe from Vial A. | [ ] | [ ] | [ ] |
| 6. | Aspirate volume of air equal to the medication dose from second medication (Vial B).  Inject air into Vial B. | [ ] | [ ] | [ ] |
| 7. | Invert Vial B and withdraw required volume of medication into syringe. | [ ] | [ ] | [ ] |
| 8. | Expel all air bubbles and withdraw needle from Vial B. Remove needle. Dispose properly. | [ ] | [ ] | [ ] |
| 9. | Attach new sterile needle to syringe. | [ ] | [ ] | [ ] |
| 10. | Determine what total combined volume of medication measures on syringe scale. | [ ] | [ ] | [ ] |
| 11. | Insert needle into Vial A, invert vial, and carefully withdraw required volume of medication. | [ ] | [ ] | [ ] |
| 12. | Withdraw needle from  Vial A. | [ ] | [ ] | [ ] |
| 13. | Check medication and dosage before returning or discarding vials. | [ ] | [ ] | [ ] |
| 14. | Wash hands. | [ ] | [ ] | [ ] |

E = Excels;  S = Satisfactory;  U = Unsatisfactory

COMMENTS:

[ ] Pass  [ ] Fail

Student's Signature_____ Date_____

Instructor's Signature_____ Date _____

© 1992 J.B. Lippincott Company, Fundamentals of Nursing:  Human Health and Function

28

# PROCEDURE 24-2B
## DRAWING UP TWO MEDICATIONS IN A SYRINGE
### MODIFICATION FOR INSULIN

|  |  | E | S | U |
|---|---|---|---|---|
| 1. | Wash hands. | [ ] | [ ] | [ ] |
| 2. | Gently rotate vials between palms of hands to mix solutions of insulin in suspension. | [ ] | [ ] | [ ] |
| 3. | Cleanse tops of both vials with antiseptic. | [ ] | [ ] | [ ] |
| 4. | With syringe, aspirate volume of air equal to medication dose from first medication (Vial A). | [ ] | [ ] | [ ] |
| 5. | Inject air into Vial A, being careful that needle does not touch solution. | [ ] | [ ] | [ ] |
| 6. | Remove syringe from Vial A. | [ ] | [ ] | [ ] |
| 7. | Aspirate volume of air equal to medication dose from second medication (Vial B). Inject air into Vial B. | [ ] | [ ] | [ ] |
| 8. | Invert Vial B and withdraw required volume of medication into syringe. | [ ] | [ ] | [ ] |
| 9. | Draw Regular Insulin into syringe first. | [ ] | [ ] | [ ] |
| 10. | Expel all air bubbles and withdraw needle from Vial B. | [ ] | [ ] | [ ] |
| 11. | Remove needle and dispose of properly. Attach new sterile needle to syringe. | [ ] | [ ] | [ ] |
| 12. | Determine what total combined volume of medication measures on syringe scale. | [ ] | [ ] | [ ] |
| 13. | Insert needle into Vial A, invert vial, and carefully withdraw required volume of medication. | [ ] | [ ] | [ ] |
| 14. | Withdraw needle from Vial A. | [ ] | [ ] | [ ] |
| 15. | Check medication and dosage before returning or discarding vials. | [ ] | [ ] | [ ] |
| 16. | Have another nurse cross-check insulin dosage against physician's order while drawing up medication. | [ ] | [ ] | [ ] |
| 16. | Wash hands. | [ ] | [ ] | [ ] |

E = Excels;  S = Satisfactory;  U = Unsatisfactory

COMMENTS:

[ ] Pass  [ ] Fail

Student's Signature_____ Date_____

Instructor's Signature_____ Date _____

© 1992 J.B. Lippincott Company, Fundamentals of Nursing: Human Health and Function

## PROCEDURE 24-3A
## ADMINISTERING SUBCUTANEOUS INJECTIONS

|  |  | E | S | U |
|---|---|---|---|---|
| 1. | Check medication order. | [ ] | [ ] | [ ] |
| 2. | Wash hands. | [ ] | [ ] | [ ] |
| 3. | Assemble needle and syringe. | [ ] | [ ] | [ ] |
| 4. | Remove needle guard. | [ ] | [ ] | [ ] |
| 5. | Vials: | | | |
|  | a. Rotate vial between palms to disperse medication. | [ ] | [ ] | [ ] |
|  | b. Cleanse top of medication vial with alcohol swab. | [ ] | [ ] | [ ] |
|  | c. Pull back barrel on syringe to an amount of air equal to volume of medication dosage to be withdrawn. | [ ] | [ ] | [ ] |
|  | d. Insert needle into vial and inject air. | [ ] | [ ] | [ ] |
|  | e. Invert vial and withdraw desired volume of medication. | [ ] | [ ] | [ ] |
| 6. | Ampules: | | | |
|  | a. Flick upper stem of ampule with fingernail several times. | [ ] | [ ] | [ ] |
|  | b. Wrap sterile gauze or alcohol wipe around ampule neck and break off top at neck by snapping it away from you. | [ ] | [ ] | [ ] |
|  | c. Insert needle into ampule and withdraw required dosage of medication.  Hold on side to withdraw all medication. | [ ] | [ ] | [ ] |
|  | d. Dispose of used ampule in appropriate container. | [ ] | [ ] | [ ] |
| 7. | Cover needle with guard. | [ ] | [ ] | [ ] |
| 8. | If using filter needle instead of regular needle to draw up medication, replace by regular subcutaneous needle before injecting patient. | [ ] | [ ] | [ ] |
| 9. | Recheck drug and dosage against medication order or card for accuracy. | [ ] | [ ] | [ ] |
| 10. | Explain procedure to patient and identify patient by name and identification bracelet. | [ ] | [ ] | [ ] |
| 11. | Select injection site that is free from tenderness, swelling, scarring, inflammation. | [ ] | [ ] | [ ] |
| 12. | Don glove on nondominant hand, if required by agency policy. | [ ] | [ ] | [ ] |
| 13. | Cleanse site with antiseptic swab in circular motion from center outward.  Allow area to dry thoroughly. | [ ] | [ ] | [ ] |
| 14. | Remove needle cap and expel air bubbles from syringe.  Hold syringe in dominant hand. | [ ] | [ ] | [ ] |
| 15. | Place nondominant hand on either side of injection site. Spread or pinch skin to stabilize site. | [ ] | [ ] | [ ] |
| 16. | Hold syringe between thumb and forefinger of dominant hand. Inject needle quickly at a 45 to 90 degree angle depending on amount of adipose tissue.  Release pinched skin. | [ ] | [ ] | [ ] |
| 17. | Aspirate by slowly pulling back on plunger.  If blood appears in syringe, withdraw needle, discard syringe and prepare new injection. | [ ] | [ ] | [ ] |

*(continued)*

© 1992 J.B. Lippincott Company, Fundamentals of Nursing: Human Health and Function

## 24-3A:  Administering Subcutaneous Injections *(Continued)*

|  |  | E | S | U |
|---|---|---|---|---|
| 18. | If no blood appears, inject medication with slow even pressure. | [ ] | [ ] | [ ] |
| 19. | Remove needle quickly while pressing antiseptic swab over site. | [ ] | [ ] | [ ] |
| 20. | Gently massage site with antiseptic swab if not contraindicated. | [ ] | [ ] | [ ] |
| 22. | Dispose of <u>uncapped</u> needle and syringe in appropriate container. | [ ] | [ ] | [ ] |
| 23. | Wash hands. | [ ] | [ ] | [ ] |
| 24. | Record according to agency protocol. | [ ] | [ ] | [ ] |

E = Excels;  S = Satisfactory;  U = Unsatisfactory

COMMENTS:

[ ] Pass  [ ] Fail

Student's Signature_____ Date_____

Instructor's Signature_____ Date _____

© 1992 J.B. Lippincott Company, Fundamentals of Nursing:  Human Health and Function

# PROCEDURE 24-3B
## ADMINISTERING SUBCUTANEOUS HEPARIN

|  | E | S | U |
|---|---|---|---|
| 1. Check medication order. | [ ] | [ ] | [ ] |
| 2. Wash hands. | [ ] | [ ] | [ ] |
| 3. Assemble needle and syringe. | [ ] | [ ] | [ ] |
| 4. Remove needle guard. | [ ] | [ ] | [ ] |
| 5. Vials: |  |  |  |
| a. Rotate vial between palms to disperse medication. | [ ] | [ ] | [ ] |
| b. Cleanse top of medication vial with alcohol swab. | [ ] | [ ] | [ ] |
| c. Pull back barrel on syringe to an amount of air equal to volume of medication dosage to be withdrawn. | [ ] | [ ] | [ ] |
| d. Insert needle into vial and inject air. | [ ] | [ ] | [ ] |
| e. Invert vial and withdraw desired volume of medication. | [ ] | [ ] | [ ] |
| 6. Ampules: |  |  |  |
| a. Flick upper stem of ampule with fingernail several times. | [ ] | [ ] | [ ] |
| b. Wrap sterile gauze or alcohol wipe around ampule neck and break off top at neck by snapping it away from you. | [ ] | [ ] | [ ] |
| c. Insert needle into ampule and withdraw required dosage of medication. Hold on side to withdraw all medication. | [ ] | [ ] | [ ] |
| d. Dispose of used ampule in appropriate container. | [ ] | [ ] | [ ] |
| 7. Cover needle with guard. | [ ] | [ ] | [ ] |
| 8. If using filter needle instead of regular needle to draw up medication, replace by regular subcutaneous needle before injecting patient. | [ ] | [ ] | [ ] |
| 9. Recheck drug and dosage against medication order or card for accuracy. | [ ] | [ ] | [ ] |
| 10. Explain procedure to patient and identify patient by name and identification bracelet. | [ ] | [ ] | [ ] |
| 11. Select injection site on abdomen on either side of umbilicus that is free from tenderness, swelling, scarring, inflammation. | [ ] | [ ] | [ ] |
| 12. Don glove on nondominant hand, if required by agency policy. | [ ] | [ ] | [ ] |
| 13. Cleanse site with antiseptic swab in circular motion from center outward. Allow area to dry thoroughly. | [ ] | [ ] | [ ] |
| 14. Remove needle cap and expel air bubbles from syringe. Hold syringe in dominant hand. | [ ] | [ ] | [ ] |
| 15. Place nondominant hand on either side of injection site. Spread to stabilize site. | [ ] | [ ] | [ ] |
| 16. Hold syringe between thumb and forefinger of dominant hand. Inject needle quickly at a 45 to 90 degree angle depending on amount of adipose tissue. | [ ] | [ ] | [ ] |
| 17. Inject medication with slow even pressure. | [ ] | [ ] | [ ] |
| 18. Remove needle quickly while pressing antiseptic swab over site. | [ ] | [ ] | [ ] |
| 19. Assist patient to position of comfort. | [ ] | [ ] | [ ] |

*(continued)*

© 1992 J.B. Lippincott Company, Fundamentals of Nursing: Human Health and Function

**24-3B: Administering Subcutaneous Heparin** *(Continued)*

|  | E | S | U |
|---|---|---|---|
| 20. Dispose of <u>uncapped</u> needle and syringe in appropriate container. | [ ] | [ ] | [ ] |
| 21. Wash hands. | [ ] | [ ] | [ ] |

E = Excels;  S = Satisfactory;  U = Unsatisfactory

COMMENTS:

[ ] Pass  [ ] Fail

Student's Signature_____ Date_____

Instructor's Signature_____ Date _____

© 1992 J.B. Lippincott Company, Fundamentals of Nursing:  Human Health and Function

# PROCEDURE 24-4A
## ADMINISTERING INTRAMUSCULAR INJECTIONS

| | E | S | U |
|---|---|---|---|
| 1. Check medication order. | [ ] | [ ] | [ ] |
| 2. Wash hands. | [ ] | [ ] | [ ] |
| 3. Assemble needle and syringe. | [ ] | [ ] | [ ] |
| 4. Remove needle guard. | [ ] | [ ] | [ ] |
| 5. Vials: | | | |
|     a. Rotate vial between palms to disperse medication. | [ ] | [ ] | [ ] |
|     b. Cleanse top of medication vial with alcohol swab. | [ ] | [ ] | [ ] |
|     c. Pull back barrel on syringe to an amount of air equal to volume of medication dosage to be withdrawn. | [ ] | [ ] | [ ] |
|     d. Insert needle into vial and inject air. | [ ] | [ ] | [ ] |
|     e. Invert vial and withdraw desired volume of medication. | [ ] | [ ] | [ ] |
| 6. Ampules: | | | |
|     a. Flick upper stem of ampule with fingernail several times. | [ ] | [ ] | [ ] |
|     b. Wrap sterile gauze or alcohol wipe around ampule neck and break off top at neck by snapping it away from you. | [ ] | [ ] | [ ] |
|     c. Insert needle into ampule and withdraw required dosage of medication.  Hold on side to withdraw all medication. | [ ] | [ ] | [ ] |
|     d. Dispose of used ampule in appropriate container. | [ ] | [ ] | [ ] |
| 7. Cover needle with guard. | [ ] | [ ] | [ ] |
| 8. If using filter needle instead of regular needle to draw up medication, replace by regular intramuscular needle before injecting patient. | [ ] | [ ] | [ ] |
| 9. If medication is known to be irritating to tissues, replace needle after withdrawing medication. | [ ] | [ ] | [ ] |
| 10. Recheck drug and dosage against medication order or card for accuracy. | [ ] | [ ] | [ ] |
| 11. Explain procedure to patient and identify patient by name and identification bracelet. | [ ] | [ ] | [ ] |
| 12. Select appropriate injection site by inspecting muscle size and integrity.  Consider volume of medication to be injected. | [ ] | [ ] | [ ] |
| 13. Assist patient to a comfortable position and expose only the area to be injected. | [ ] | [ ] | [ ] |
| 14. Use anatomic landmarks to locate exact injection site. | [ ] | [ ] | [ ] |
| 15. Don glove on nondominant hand, if required by agency policy. | [ ] | [ ] | [ ] |
| 16. Cleanse site with antiseptic swab, wiping from center of site and rotating outward. | [ ] | [ ] | [ ] |
| 17. Remove needle cover. | [ ] | [ ] | [ ] |
| 18. Expel air bubbles from syringe. | [ ] | [ ] | [ ] |
| 19. Hold syringe between thumb and forefinger of dominant hand like a dart. | [ ] | [ ] | [ ] |

*(continued)*

© 1992 J.B. Lippincott Company, Fundamentals of Nursing:  Human Health and Function

## 24-4A: Administering Intramuscular Injections *(Continued)*

|  | E | S | U |
|---|---|---|---|
| 20. Spread skin at the side with nondominant hand. If small muscle mass, pinch skin. | [ ] | [ ] | [ ] |
| 22. Stabilize syringe barrel by grasping with nondominant hand. Aspirate slowly by pulling back on plunger with dominant hand. If no blood appears, inject medication slowly. | [ ] | [ ] | [ ] |
| 23. If blood appears, remove needle, dispose of syringe, and prepare new medication. | [ ] | [ ] | [ ] |
| 24. Withdraw needle while pressing antiseptic swab above site. | [ ] | [ ] | [ ] |
| 25. Gently massage site. | [ ] | [ ] | [ ] |
| 26. Dispose of uncapped needle and syringe in proper receptacle. | [ ] | [ ] | [ ] |
| 27. Wash hands. | [ ] | [ ] | [ ] |
| 28. Record medication and patient response according to agency protocol. | [ ] | [ ] | [ ] |

E = Excels;  S = Satisfactory;  U = Unsatisfactory

**COMMENTS:**

[ ] Pass  [ ] Fail

Student's Signature_____ Date_____

Instructor's Signature_____ Date _____

© 1992 J.B. Lippincott Company, Fundamentals of Nursing:  Human Health and Function

# PROCEDURE 24-4B
## ADMINISTERING INTRAMUSCULAR INJECTIONS
### AIR LOCK INJECTION TECHNIQUE

|  | E | S | U |
|---|---|---|---|
| 1. Check medication order. | [ ] | [ ] | [ ] |
| 2. Wash hands. | [ ] | [ ] | [ ] |
| 3. Assemble needle and syringe. | [ ] | [ ] | [ ] |
| 4. Remove needle guard. | [ ] | [ ] | [ ] |
| 5. Vials: | | | |
| a. Rotate vial between palms to disperse medication. | [ ] | [ ] | [ ] |
| b. Cleanse top of medication vial with alcohol swab. | [ ] | [ ] | [ ] |
| c. Pull back barrel on syringe to an amount of air equal to volume of medication dosage to be withdrawn. | [ ] | [ ] | [ ] |
| d. Insert needle into vial and inject air. | [ ] | [ ] | [ ] |
| e. Invert vial and withdraw desired volume of medication. Expel all air. | [ ] | [ ] | [ ] |
| 6. Ampules: | | | |
| a. Flick upper stem of ampule with fingernail several times. | [ ] | [ ] | [ ] |
| b. Wrap sterile gauze or alcohol wipe around ampule neck and break off top at neck by snapping it away from you. | [ ] | [ ] | [ ] |
| c. Insert needle into ampule and withdraw required dosage of medication. Hold on side to withdraw all medication. Expel all excess air. | [ ] | [ ] | [ ] |
| d. Dispose of used ampule in appropriate container. | [ ] | [ ] | [ ] |
| 7. Note there is approximately 0.2 mL more solution than necessary for accurate dosage. Expel the volume of solution not required in prescribed dosage. Pull back plunger and visually inspect syringe for correct dosage. | [ ] | [ ] | [ ] |
| 8. Expel all excess air from syringe, leaving only 0.2 mL air. | [ ] | [ ] | [ ] |
| 9. Cover needle with guard. | [ ] | [ ] | [ ] |
| 10. If using filter needle instead of regular needle to draw up medication, replace by regular intramuscular needle before injecting patient. | [ ] | [ ] | [ ] |
| 11. If medication is known to be irritating to tissues, replace needle after withdrawing medication. | [ ] | [ ] | [ ] |
| 12. Recheck drug and dosage against medication order or card for accuracy. | [ ] | [ ] | [ ] |
| 13. Explain procedure to patient and identify patient by name and identification bracelet. | [ ] | [ ] | [ ] |
| 14. Select appropriate injection site by inspecting muscle size and integrity. Consider volume of medication to be injected. | [ ] | [ ] | [ ] |
| 15. Assist patient to a comfortable position and expose only the area to be injected. | [ ] | [ ] | [ ] |

*(continued)*

© 1992 J.B. Lippincott Company, Fundamentals of Nursing: Human Health and Function

**24-4B: Administering Intramuscular Injections**
**Air Lock Injection Technique** *(Continued)*

|  | E | S | U |
|---|---|---|---|
| 16. Use anatomic landmarks to locate exact injection site. | [ ] | [ ] | [ ] |
| 17. Don glove on nondominant hand, if required by agency policy. | [ ] | [ ] | [ ] |
| 18. Cleanse site with antiseptic swab, wiping from center of site and rotating outward. | [ ] | [ ] | [ ] |
| 19. Remove needle cover. | [ ] | [ ] | [ ] |
| 20. Expel air bubbles from syringe. | [ ] | [ ] | [ ] |
| 21. Hold syringe between thumb and forefinger of dominant hand like a dart. | [ ] | [ ] | [ ] |
| 22. Spread skin at the side with nondominant hand. If small muscle mass, pinch skin. | [ ] | [ ] | [ ] |
| 23. Insert needle quickly at a 90 degree angle to floor. | [ ] | [ ] | [ ] |
| 24. Stabilize syringe barrel by grasping with nondominant hand. Aspirate slowly by pulling back on plunger with dominant hand. If no blood appears, inject medication slowly. | [ ] | [ ] | [ ] |
| 25. If blood appears, remove needle, dispose of syringe, and prepare new medication. | [ ] | [ ] | [ ] |
| 26. Withdraw needle while pressing antiseptic swab above site. | [ ] | [ ] | [ ] |
| 27. Gently massage site. | [ ] | [ ] | [ ] |
| 28. Dispose of uncapped needle and syringe in proper receptacle. | [ ] | [ ] | [ ] |
| 29. Wash hands. | [ ] | [ ] | [ ] |
| 30. Record medication and patient response according to agency protocol. | [ ] | [ ] | [ ] |

E = Excels;  S = Satisfactory;  U = Unsatisfactory

COMMENTS:

[ ] Pass  [ ] Fail

Student's Signature_____  Date_____

Instructor's Signature_____  Date _____

© 1992 J.B. Lippincott Company, Fundamentals of Nursing: Human Health and Function

## PROCEDURE 24-4C
# ADMINISTERING INTRAMUSCULAR INJECTIONS
### Z-TRACK INJECTIONS

| | E | S | U |
|---|---|---|---|
| 1. Check medication order. | [ ] | [ ] | [ ] |
| 2. Wash hands. | [ ] | [ ] | [ ] |
| 3. Assemble needle and syringe. | [ ] | [ ] | [ ] |
| 4. Remove needle guard. | [ ] | [ ] | [ ] |
| 5. Vials: | | | |
| a. Rotate vial between palms to disperse medication. | [ ] | [ ] | [ ] |
| b. Cleanse top of medication vial with alcohol swab. | [ ] | [ ] | [ ] |
| c. Pull back barrel on syringe to an amount of air equal to volume of medication dosage to be withdrawn. | [ ] | [ ] | [ ] |
| d. Insert needle into vial and inject air. | [ ] | [ ] | [ ] |
| e. Invert vial and withdraw desired volume of medication. Expel all excess air. | [ ] | [ ] | [ ] |
| 6. Ampules: | | | |
| a. Flick upper stem of ampule with fingernail several times. | [ ] | [ ] | [ ] |
| b. Wrap sterile gauze or alcohol wipe around ampule neck and break off top at neck by snapping it away from you. | [ ] | [ ] | [ ] |
| c. Insert needle into ampule and withdraw required dosage of medication. Hold on side to withdraw all medication. Expel all excess air. | [ ] | [ ] | [ ] |
| d. Dispose of used ampule in appropriate container. | [ ] | [ ] | [ ] |
| 7. Note there is approximately 0.2 mL more solution than necessary for accurate dosage. Expel the volume of solution not required in prescribed dosage. Pull back plunger and visually inspect syringe for correct dosage. | [ ] | [ ] | [ ] |
| 8. Expel all excess air from syringe, leaving only 0.2 mL air. | [ ] | [ ] | [ ] |
| 9. Cover needle with guard. | [ ] | [ ] | [ ] |
| 10. If using filter needle instead of regular needle to draw up medication, replace by regular intramuscular needle before injecting patient. | [ ] | [ ] | [ ] |
| 11. If medication is known to be irritating to tissues, replace needle after withdrawing medication. | [ ] | [ ] | [ ] |
| 12. Recheck drug and dosage against medication order or card for accuracy. | [ ] | [ ] | [ ] |
| 13. Explain procedure to patient and identify patient by name and identification bracelet. | [ ] | [ ] | [ ] |
| 14. Select appropriate injection site by inspecting muscle size and integrity. Consider volume of medication to be injected. | [ ] | [ ] | [ ] |
| 15. Assist patient to a comfortable position and expose only the area to be injected. | [ ] | [ ] | [ ] |

*(continued)*

© 1992 J.B. Lippincott Company, Fundamentals of Nursing: Human Health and Function

**24-4C:** **Administering Intramuscular Injections**
**Z-Track Injections** *(Continued)*

|  | E | S | U |
|---|---|---|---|
| 16. Use anatomic landmarks to locate exact injection site. | [ ] | [ ] | [ ] |
| 17. Don glove on nondominant hand, if required by agency policy. | [ ] | [ ] | [ ] |
| 18. Cleanse site with antiseptic swab, wiping from center of site and rotating outward. | [ ] | [ ] | [ ] |
| 19. Remove needle cover. | [ ] | [ ] | [ ] |
| 20. Expel air bubbles from syringe. | [ ] | [ ] | [ ] |
| 21. Hold syringe between thumb and forefinger of dominant hand like a dart. | [ ] | [ ] | [ ] |
| 22. Pull skin and subcutaneous tissue about 1 to 1.5 inches to one side of selected site. | [ ] | [ ] | [ ] |
| 23. Insert needle quickly at a 90 degree angle. | [ ] | [ ] | [ ] |
| 24. Stabilize syringe barrel by grasping with nondominant hand. Aspirate slowly by pulling back on plunger with dominant hand. If no blood appears, inject medication slowly while continuing traction on skin. | [ ] | [ ] | [ ] |
| 25. If blood appears, remove needle, dispose of syringe, and prepare new medication. | [ ] | [ ] | [ ] |
| 26. Leave needle inserted an additional 10 seconds. Withdraw needle while pressing antiseptic swab above site. Release traction on skin. | [ ] | [ ] | [ ] |
| 27. Gently massage site. | [ ] | [ ] | [ ] |
| 28. Dispose of uncapped needle and syringe in proper receptacle. | [ ] | [ ] | [ ] |
| 29. Wash hands. | [ ] | [ ] | [ ] |
| 30. Record medication and patient response according to agency protocol. | [ ] | [ ] | [ ] |

E = Excels;  S = Satisfactory;  U = Unsatisfactory

COMMENTS:

[ ] Pass  [ ] Fail

Student's Signature_____  Date_____

Instructor's Signature_____  Date _____

© 1992 J.B. Lippincott Company, Fundamentals of Nursing: Human Health and Function

## PROCEDURE 24-5A
## ADMINISTERING IV MEDICATIONS USING INTERMITTENT
### INFUSION TECHNIQUE

|  |  | E | S | U |
|---|---|---|---|---|
| 1. | Wash hands. | [ ] | [ ] | [ ] |
| 2. | Connect infusion tubing to medication container. | [ ] | [ ] | [ ] |
| 3. | Connect capped, sterile needle to end of infusion set. | [ ] | [ ] | [ ] |
| 4. | Confirm patient's identity by asking name, and looking at identiband. | [ ] | [ ] | [ ] |
| 5. | Hang medication bag at or above level of primary IV solution. | [ ] | [ ] | [ ] |
| 6. | Wipe injection port, nearest IV insertion site, on primary IV tubing with antiseptic. | [ ] | [ ] | [ ] |
| 7. | Remove needle cover from medication tubing and insert injection port of primary IV line. Secure with tape. | [ ] | [ ] | [ ] |
| 8. | If IV medication is not compatible with primary IV solution, clamp primary IV tubing above injection port, insert needle with 20 mL syringe of NaCl and flush IV line. Remove needle. Insert needle attached to medication tubing and secure with tape. | [ ] | [ ] | [ ] |
| 9. | Regulate flow of medication solution. Infuse over 20 to 60 minutes according to pharmacy directives. Monitor periodically. | [ ] | [ ] | [ ] |
| 10. | When medication has infused, turn off flow clamp. Regulate primary infusion as necessary. | [ ] | [ ] | [ ] |
| 11. | Discard medication solution container, tubing, and needle or leave hanging with needle covered for future use, according to agency policy. | [ ] | [ ] | [ ] |
| 12. | Wash hands. | [ ] | [ ] | [ ] |
| 13. | Document medication administration and add IV volume to IV intake. | [ ] | [ ] | [ ] |

E = Excels;  S = Satisfactory;  U = Unsatisfactory

COMMENTS:

[ ] Pass  [ ] Fail

Student's Signature_____ Date_____

Instructor's Signature_____ Date _____

© 1992 J.B. Lippincott Company, Fundamentals of Nursing: Human Health and Function

## PROCEDURE 24-5B
# ADMINISTERING IV MEDICATIONS USING INTERMITTENT
## INFUSION TECHNIQUE
## USING A HEPARIN LOCK

|  |  | E | S | U |
|---|---|---|---|---|
| 1. | Wash hands. | [ ] | [ ] | [ ] |
| 2. | Connect infusion tubing to medication container. | [ ] | [ ] | [ ] |
| 3. | Connect capped, sterile needle to end of infusion set. | [ ] | [ ] | [ ] |
| 4. | Confirm patient's identity by asking name, and looking at identiband. | [ ] | [ ] | [ ] |
| 5. | Hang medication bag at or above level of primary IV solution. | [ ] | [ ] | [ ] |
| 6. | Wipe injection port, nearest IV insertion site, on primary IV tubing with antiseptic. | [ ] | [ ] | [ ] |
| 7. | Insert needle of the 3 mL NaCl syringe into port. Aspirate for blood return. | [ ] | [ ] | [ ] |
| 8. | Inject 2 to 3 mL of NaCl without forcing solution. | [ ] | [ ] | [ ] |
| 9. | Remove needle and discard in appropriate receptacle. | [ ] | [ ] | [ ] |
| 10. | Insert needle of medication tubing into injection port. Secure and regulate flow according to pharmacy directive. Monitor periodically. | [ ] | [ ] | [ ] |
| 11. | When medication has infused, turn off clamp and remove needle. | [ ] | [ ] | [ ] |
| 12. | Cleanse port. | [ ] | [ ] | [ ] |
| 13. | Insert needle of second NaCl syringe and inject 2 to 3 mL NaCl. Discard. | [ ] | [ ] | [ ] |
| 14. | Insert needle of heparin flush solution. Inject slowly. Remove needle and discard. | [ ] | [ ] | [ ] |
| 15. | Wash hands. | [ ] | [ ] | [ ] |
| 16. | Document medication administration, heparin flush, and add IV volume to IV intake. | [ ] | [ ] | [ ] |

E = Excels;  S = Satisfactory;  U = Unsatisfactory

COMMENTS:

[ ] Pass  [ ] Fail

Student's Signature_____ Date_____

Instructor's Signature_____ Date _____

© 1992 J.B. Lippincott Company, Fundamentals of Nursing: Human Health and Function

# PROCEDURE 28-1
# BATHING A PATIENT IN BED

|  |  | E | S | U |
|---|---|---|---|---|
| 1. | Close curtains around bed or shut room door. | [ ] | [ ] | [ ] |
| 2. | Help patient to use bedpan, urinal, or commode, if needed. | [ ] | [ ] | [ ] |
| 3. | Close window and doors to decrease drafts. | [ ] | [ ] | [ ] |
| 4. | Wash your hands. | [ ] | [ ] | [ ] |
| 5. | Raise bed to high position. Lock siderail up on opposite side of bed from your work. | [ ] | [ ] | [ ] |
| 6. | Remove top sheet and bed spread and place bath blanket on patient. Help patient move closer to you, and remove gown. | [ ] | [ ] | [ ] |
| 7. | If reusing top linen, place it on back of chair; otherwise, place in laundry bag. | [ ] | [ ] | [ ] |
| 8. | If patient has an IV line, remove gown from arm, lower IV container, and slide it through gown with tubing. Rehang IV container and check flow rate. | [ ] | [ ] | [ ] |
| 9. | Lay towel across patient's chest. | [ ] | [ ] | [ ] |
| 10. | Wet washcloth and fold around your finger to make a mitt. | [ ] | [ ] | [ ] |
|  | a. Fold washcloth in thirds. |  |  |  |
|  | b. Straighten washcloth to take out wrinkles. |  |  |  |
|  | c. Fold washcloth over to fit hand. |  |  |  |
|  | d. Tuck loose ends under edge of washcloth on palm. |  |  |  |
| 11. | Cleanse eyes with water only, wiping from inner to outer canthus. Use separate corner of mitt for each eye. | [ ] | [ ] | [ ] |
| 12. | Determine if patient would like soap used on face. Wash face, neck, and ears. | [ ] | [ ] | [ ] |
| 13. | Fold bath blanket off arm away from you. Place towel lengthwise under arm. Wash, rinse, and dry the arm using long firm stroked from fingers toward axilla. Wash axilla. | [ ] | [ ] | [ ] |
| 14. | (Optional) Place bath towel on bed and put wash basin on it. Immerse patient's hand and allow to soak for several minutes. Wash, rinse, and dry hand well. Repeat on other side. Apply lotion. | [ ] | [ ] | [ ] |
| 15. | Repeat for arm and hand nearest you. | [ ] | [ ] | [ ] |
| 16. | Apply deodorant or powder according to patient preferences. Avoid excessive use of powder or inhalation of powder. | [ ] | [ ] | [ ] |
| 17. | Assess temperature of bath water and change water if necessary. If you leave bedside, lock siderails up to prevent accidental falls. | [ ] | [ ] | [ ] |
| 18. | Place bath towel over chest. Fold bath blanket down to below umbilicus. | [ ] | [ ] | [ ] |

*(continued)*

© 1992 J.B. Lippincott Company, Fundamentals of Nursing: Human Health and Function

## 28-1: Bathing A Patient In Bed *(Continued)*

|  | E | S | U |
|---|---|---|---|
| 19. Lift bath towel off chest and bathe chest and abdomen with mitted hand using long, firm strokes. Give special attention to skin under breasts and any other skin folds, if patient is overweight. Rinse and dry well. | [ ] | [ ] | [ ] |
| 20. Help patient don clean gown. | [ ] | [ ] | [ ] |
| 21. Expose leg away from you by folding over bath blanket. Be careful to keep perineum covered. | [ ] | [ ] | [ ] |
| 22. Lift leg and place bath towel lengthwise under leg. Wash, rinse and dry leg using long, firm strokes from ankle to thigh. | [ ] | [ ] | [ ] |
| 23. Wash feet or place in basin of water as for hands. Rinse and dry well. Pay special attention to space between toes. | [ ] | [ ] | [ ] |
| 24. Repeat for other leg and foot. | [ ] | [ ] | [ ] |
| 25. Assess bath water for warmth. Change water if necessary. | [ ] | [ ] | [ ] |
| 26. Assist patient to side-lying position. Place bath towel alongside of back and buttocks to protect linen. Wash, rinse, and dry back and buttocks. Give backrub with powder or lotion. | [ ] | [ ] | [ ] |
| 27. Assist to supine position. Assess if patient can wash genitals and perineal area independently. If unable, drape with bath blanket so that only genitals are exposed. Don disposable, clean gloves, wash, rinse, and dry genitalia and perineum. | [ ] | [ ] | [ ] |
| 28. Apply powder, lotion, cologne according to patient preference. | [ ] | [ ] | [ ] |
| 29. Assist with hair and mouth care. | [ ] | [ ] | [ ] |
| 30. Make bed with clean linen. | [ ] | [ ] | [ ] |
| 31. Clean equipment and return to appropriate storage area. | [ ] | [ ] | [ ] |
| 32. Wash your hands. | [ ] | [ ] | [ ] |
| 33. Record significant observations. | [ ] | [ ] | [ ] |

E = Excels;  S = Satisfactory;  U = Unsatisfactory

COMMENTS:

[ ] Pass  [ ] Fail

Student's Signature_____ Date_____

Instructor's Signature_____ Date _____

© 1992 J.B. Lippincott Company, Fundamentals of Nursing: Human Health and Function

# PROCEDURE 28-2
## ASSISTING WITH THE BATH OR SHOWER

|  |  | E | S | U |
|---|---|---|---|---|
| 1. | Place towel or disposable bath mat on floor by tub or shower. | [ ] | [ ] | [ ] |
| 2. | Help patient to bathroom. | [ ] | [ ] | [ ] |
| 3. | Place "occupied" sign on bathroom door. | [ ] | [ ] | [ ] |
| 4. | Fill bathtub halfway with warm water (105° F). Test water or have patient test water. If taking shower, turn shower on and adjust temperature. | [ ] | [ ] | [ ] |
| 5. | Help patient into shower or tub, providing necessary assistance. | [ ] | [ ] | [ ] |
| 6. | Check on patient within 15 minutes. Wash any areas he or she cannot reach. | [ ] | [ ] | [ ] |
| 7. | Help patient out of tub or shower. Assist with drying. | [ ] | [ ] | [ ] |
| 8. | If patient is unsteady, drain water before getting patient out of tub to prevent falls. | [ ] | [ ] | [ ] |
| 9. | Assist patient with dressing and grooming. | [ ] | [ ] | [ ] |
| 10. | Help patient to room. | [ ] | [ ] | [ ] |
| 11. | Return to bathroom to clean tub or shower according to agency policy. Discard soiled linen. Place "unoccupied" sign on door. | [ ] | [ ] | [ ] |

E = Excels;  S = Satisfactory;  U = Unsatisfactory

COMMENTS:

[ ] Pass  [ ] Fail

Student's Signature_____ Date_____

Instructor's Signature_____ Date _____

© 1992 J.B. Lippincott Company, Fundamentals of Nursing: Human Health and Function

44

## PROCEDURE 28-3
## MASSAGING THE BACK

|  | E | S | U |
|---|---|---|---|
| 1. Help patient to side-lying or prone position. | [ ] | [ ] | [ ] |
| 2. Expose back, shoulders, upper arms, and sacral area. Cover remainder of body with bath blanket. | [ ] | [ ] | [ ] |
| 3. Wash hands in warm water. Warm lotion by holding container under running warm water. | [ ] | [ ] | [ ] |
| 4. Pour small amount of lotion into palms. | [ ] | [ ] | [ ] |
| 5. Begin massage in sacral area with circular motion. Move hands upward to shoulders, massaging over scapulae in smooth, firm strokes. Without removing hands from skin, continue in smooth strokes to upper arms and down sides of back to iliac crest. Continue for 3 to 5 minutes. | [ ] | [ ] | [ ] |
| 6. While massaging, assess for whitish or reddened areas that do not disappear, and broken skin areas. | [ ] | [ ] | [ ] |
| 7. If additional stimulation is desired, petrissage (kneading) over shoulders and gluteal area and tapotement (tapping) up and down spine is done. | [ ] | [ ] | [ ] |
| 8. End massage with long, continuous, stroking movements. | [ ] | [ ] | [ ] |
| 9. Pat excess lubricant dry with towel. Retie gown and assist to comfortable position. | [ ] | [ ] | [ ] |
| 10. Wash hands. | [ ] | [ ] | [ ] |

E = Excels;  S = Satisfactory;  U = Unsatisfactory

COMMENTS:

[ ] Pass  [ ] Fail

Student's Signature_____ Date_____

Instructor's Signature_____ Date_____

© 1992 J.B. Lippincott Company, Fundamentals of Nursing: Human Health and Function

## PROCEDURE 28-4
## PERFORMING FOOT AND NAIL CARE

|  | E | S | U |
|---|---|---|---|
| 1. Wash hands. | [ ] | [ ] | [ ] |
| 2. Help patient to chair if possible. Elevate head of bed for bedridden patient. | [ ] | [ ] | [ ] |
| 3. Remove colored nail polish if patient is scheduled for surgery. Review agency policy to determine if patient may wear clear nail polish. | [ ] | [ ] | [ ] |
| 4. Fill wash basin with warm water (100-104° F). Place waterproof pad under basin. Soak patient's hands or feet in basin. | [ ] | [ ] | [ ] |
| 5. Place call bell within reach. Allow hands or feet to soak for 10 to 20 minutes. | [ ] | [ ] | [ ] |
| 6. Dry hand or foot that has been soaking. Rewarm water and allow other extremity to soak while you work on the softened nails. | [ ] | [ ] | [ ] |
| 7. Gently clean under nails with orange stick. If nails are thickened and yellow, patient may have fungal infection. Don disposable clean gloves. | [ ] | [ ] | [ ] |
| 8. Beginning with large toe or thumb, clip nail straight across. Shape nail with file. File rather than cut nails of patient with diabetes or circulatory problems. | [ ] | [ ] | [ ] |
| 9. Refer patient with severely hypertrophied nails to podiatrist or foot clinic. | [ ] | [ ] | [ ] |
| 10. Push cuticle back gently with orange stick. | [ ] | [ ] | [ ] |
| 11. Repeat procedure with other nails. | [ ] | [ ] | [ ] |
| 12. Rinse foot or hand in warm water. | [ ] | [ ] | [ ] |
| 13. Dry thoroughly with towel. | [ ] | [ ] | [ ] |
| 14. Apply lotion to hands or feet. | [ ] | [ ] | [ ] |
| 15. Help patient to comfortable position. | [ ] | [ ] | [ ] |
| 16. Remove and dispose of equipment. | [ ] | [ ] | [ ] |
| 17. Wash hands. | [ ] | [ ] | [ ] |

E = Excels;  S = Satisfactory;  U = Unsatisfactory

COMMENTS:

[ ] Pass  [ ] Fail

Student's Signature_____ Date_____

Instructor's Signature_____ Date _____

© 1992 J.B. Lippincott Company, Fundamentals of Nursing: Human Health and Function

# PROCEDURE 28-5
## SHAMPOOING HAIR OF BEDRIDDEN PATIENT

|  |  | E | S | U |
|---|---|---|---|---|
| 1. | Place waterproof pads under patient's head and shoulders and remove pillow. | [ ] | [ ] | [ ] |
| 2. | Raise bed to highest position. | [ ] | [ ] | [ ] |
| 3. | Remove any pins from hair.  Comb and brush hair thoroughly. | [ ] | [ ] | [ ] |
| 4. | Lay bed to flat position. | [ ] | [ ] | [ ] |
| 5. | Place shampooing basin under head.  Place bath towel around shoulders and folded washcloth where neck rests on basin. | [ ] | [ ] | [ ] |
| 6. | Fold bed linens down to waist.  Cover upper body with bath blanket. | [ ] | [ ] | [ ] |
| 7. | Place wash basin under spout of shampoo basin on a chair or table at the bedside. | [ ] | [ ] | [ ] |
| 8. | Place dampened washcloth over patient's eyes. | [ ] | [ ] | [ ] |
| 9. | Using water pitcher, wet hair thoroughly with warm water (approximately 110° F).  Check temperature by placing small amount of water on your wrist or with bath thermometer. | [ ] | [ ] | [ ] |
| 10. | Apply small amount of shampoo.  If needed, use hydrogen peroxide to dissolve matted blood in hair.  Reassure patient it will not bleach the hair. | [ ] | [ ] | [ ] |
| 11. | Massage scalp with fingertips while making shampoo lather.  Start at hairline and work toward neck. | [ ] | [ ] | [ ] |
| 12. | Rinse hair with warm water.  Reapply shampoo and repeat massage. | [ ] | [ ] | [ ] |
| 13. | Rinse hair thoroughly with warm water. | [ ] | [ ] | [ ] |
| 14. | Apply small amount of conditioner per patient request.  Rinse well. | [ ] | [ ] | [ ] |
| 15. | Squeeze excess moisture from hair.  Wrap bath towel around hair.  Rub to dry hair and scalp.  Use second towel if necessary. | [ ] | [ ] | [ ] |
| 16. | Remove equipment and wet towels from bed.  Place dry towel around patient's shoulders. | [ ] | [ ] | [ ] |
| 17. | Dry hair with hair dryer.  Comb and style. | [ ] | [ ] | [ ] |
| 18. | Help patient to comfortable position. | [ ] | [ ] | [ ] |
| 19. | Dispose of soiled equipment and linen. | [ ] | [ ] | [ ] |

E = Excels;  S = Satisfactory;  U = Unsatisfactory

COMMENTS:

[ ] Pass  [ ] Fail

Student's Signature_____ Date_____

Instructor's Signature_____ Date _____

© 1992 J.B. Lippincott Company, Fundamentals of Nursing:  Human Health and Function

## PROCEDURE 28-6A
## PROVIDING ORAL CARE

|  | E | S | U |
|---|---|---|---|
| 1. Wash hands. | [ ] | [ ] | [ ] |
| 2. Close bedside curtains or room door and explain procedure to patient. | [ ] | [ ] | [ ] |
| 3. Help patient to a sitting position. If patient cannot sit, help to a side-lying position. | [ ] | [ ] | [ ] |
| 4. Place towel under patient's chin. | [ ] | [ ] | [ ] |
| 5. Moisten toothbrush with water. Apply small amount of toothpaste. | [ ] | [ ] | [ ] |
| 6. Hand toothbrush to patient and don disposable gloves and brush patient's teeth as follows: | | | |
| a. Hold toothbrush at a 45 angle to gum line. | [ ] | [ ] | [ ] |
| b. Using short, vibrating motions, brush from gum line to crown of each tooth. Repeat until outside and inside of teeth and gums are cleaned. | [ ] | [ ] | [ ] |
| c. Cleanse biting surfaces by brushing with back and forth stroke. | [ ] | [ ] | [ ] |
| d. Brush tongue lightly. Avoid stimulating the gag reflex. | [ ] | [ ] | [ ] |
| 7. Have patient rinse mouth thoroughly with water and spit into emesis basin. | [ ] | [ ] | [ ] |
| 8. If tongue is heavily coated, have patient hold in mouth a half-strength hydrogen peroxide solution for a few seconds and spit out. Repeat every one to two hours. | [ ] | [ ] | [ ] |
| 9. Floss patient's teeth. | | | |
| a. Cut 10-inch piece of dental floss. Wind ends of floss around middle finger of each hand. | [ ] | [ ] | [ ] |
| b. Using index fingers to stretch the floss, move the floss up and down around and between lower teeth. Start at the back lower teeth and work around to other side. | [ ] | [ ] | [ ] |
| c. Using thumb and index fingers to stretch floss, repeat procedure on upper teeth. | [ ] | [ ] | [ ] |
| d. Have patient rinse mouth thoroughly and spit into emesis basin. | [ ] | [ ] | [ ] |
| 10. Remove basin. Dry patient's mouth. | [ ] | [ ] | [ ] |
| 11. Remove and dispose of supplies. Help patient to comfortable position. | [ ] | [ ] | [ ] |
| 12. Wash hands. | [ ] | [ ] | [ ] |

E = Excels; S = Satisfactory; U = Unsatisfactory

COMMENTS:

[ ] Pass  [ ] Fail

Student's Signature_____ Date_____

Instructor's Signature_____ Date_____

© 1992 J.B. Lippincott Company, Fundamentals of Nursing: Human Health and Function

48

**PROCEDURE 28-6B**
**PROVIDING ORAL CARE**
**VARIATION FOR UNCONSCIOUS PATIENT**

|  |  | E | S | U |
|---|---|:---:|:---:|:---:|
| 1. | Wash hands. | [ ] | [ ] | [ ] |
| 2. | Close bedside curtains or room door. | [ ] | [ ] | [ ] |
| 3. | Help to a side-lying position with head of bed lowered so saliva runs out of mouth by gravity. | [ ] | [ ] | [ ] |
| 4. | Place towel or waterproof pad under patient's chin. | [ ] | [ ] | [ ] |
| 5. | Place emesis basin against patient's mouth or have suction catheter positioned to remove secretions from mouth. | [ ] | [ ] | [ ] |
| 6. | Use padded tongue blade to open teeth gently. Leave in place between back molars without putting fingers in patient's mouth. | [ ] | [ ] | [ ] |
| 7. | Moisten toothbrush with water. Apply small amount of toothpaste. | [ ] | [ ] | [ ] |
| 8. | Don disposable gloves and brush patient's teeth as follows: | | | |
|  | a. Hold toothbrush at a 45° angle to gum line. | [ ] | [ ] | [ ] |
|  | b. Using short, vibrating motions, brush from gum line to crown of each tooth. Repeat until outside and inside of teeth and gums are cleaned. | [ ] | [ ] | [ ] |
|  | c. Cleanse biting surfaces by brushing with back and forth stroke. | [ ] | [ ] | [ ] |
|  | d. Brush tongue lightly. Avoid stimulating the gag reflex. | [ ] | [ ] | [ ] |
| 9. | Swab or suction to remove pooled secretions. Use small bulb syringe or syringe without needle to rinse oral cavity. | [ ] | [ ] | [ ] |
| 10. | Apply a thin layer of petroleum jelly to lips to prevent drying or cracking. | [ ] | [ ] | [ ] |
| 11. | Remove and dispose of supplies. Move patient to comfortable position. | [ ] | [ ] | [ ] |
| 12. | Wash hands. | [ ] | [ ] | [ ] |

E = Excels; S = Satisfactory; U = Unsatisfactory

COMMENTS:

[ ] Pass  [ ] Fail

Student's Signature_____ Date_____

Instructor's Signature_____ Date_____

© 1992 J.B. Lippincott Company, Fundamentals of Nursing: Human Health and Function

## PROCEDURE 28-7
## USING A BEDPAN

|  | E | S | U |
|---|---|---|---|

**PLACING THE BEDPAN**

|  | E | S | U |
|---|---|---|---|
| 1. Wash hands. | [ ] | [ ] | [ ] |
| 2. Close curtain around bed or shut door. | [ ] | [ ] | [ ] |
| 3. Run warm water over rim of pan; dry with towel. | [ ] | [ ] | [ ] |
| 4. Lock siderail up on opposite side of bed from which you work. | [ ] | [ ] | [ ] |
| 5. Raise bed to height appropriate for nurse. | [ ] | [ ] | [ ] |
| 6. If patient can raise buttocks and assist: | | | |
| a. Fold top linen down on nurse's side to expose patient's hips. | [ ] | [ ] | [ ] |
| b. Have patient flex knees and lift buttocks. Assist by placing your hand under sacrum, elbow on mattress, and lifting as a lever. | [ ] | [ ] | [ ] |
| c. Slide rounded smooth rim of regular bedpan under patient. If using fracture pan, slide narrow flat end under buttocks. | [ ] | [ ] | [ ] |
| 7. For patient unable to assist by raising buttocks: | | | |
| a. Lower head of bed to flat position. | [ ] | [ ] | [ ] |
| b. Fold top linens down to expose patient minimally. | [ ] | [ ] | [ ] |
| c. Help patient to roll to side-lying position. | [ ] | [ ] | [ ] |
| d. Place bedpan against buttocks and tucked down against mattress. Hold firmly in place and roll patient onto back as bedpan positions under buttocks. | [ ] | [ ] | [ ] |
| 8. Cover patient with linen. Place call bell and toilet paper within reach. | [ ] | [ ] | [ ] |
| 9. Raise head of bed 30° unless contraindicated. | [ ] | [ ] | [ ] |
| 10. Lower bed to lowest position. Place siderails up if indicated. | [ ] | [ ] | [ ] |
| 11. Wash hands. Allow patient to be alone. | [ ] | [ ] | [ ] |

**REMOVING THE BEDPAN**

|  | E | S | U |
|---|---|---|---|
| 12. Answer call bell promptly. | [ ] | [ ] | [ ] |
| 13. Place soap, wet washcloth, and towel at bedside. | [ ] | [ ] | [ ] |
| 14. Raise bed to appropriate working height for nurse. | [ ] | [ ] | [ ] |
| 15. Fold back top linens to expose patient minimally. | [ ] | [ ] | [ ] |
| 16. Put on clean disposable gloves. | [ ] | [ ] | [ ] |

*(continued)*

© 1992 J.B. Lippincott Company, Fundamentals of Nursing: Human Health and Function

28-7:  Using a Bedpan *(Continued)*

|  | E | S | U |
|---|---|---|---|
| 17. Assess if patient can wipe perineal area. If not, wipe area with several layers of toilet tissue. If specimen is to be measured or collected, dispose of soiled toilet tissue in separate receptacle, not bedpan. | [ ] | [ ] | [ ] |
| 18. For patient who can raise buttocks and assist with procedure: | | | |
| a. Lower head of bed. | [ ] | [ ] | [ ] |
| b. Have patient flex knees and lift buttocks. Assist by placing one hand under sacrum and supporting bedpan with other hand to prevent spillage. Remove bedpan and place on bedside chair. | [ ] | [ ] | [ ] |
| c. Offer soap, warm water, washcloth, and towel for patient to wash hands and/or perineal area. | [ ] | [ ] | [ ] |
| 19. For patient unable to assist by raising buttocks: | | | |
| a. Lower head of bed to flat position. | [ ] | [ ] | [ ] |
| b. Fold top linen down to expose patient minimally. | [ ] | [ ] | [ ] |
| c. Help patient to roll off bedpan and onto side. Use one hand to stabilize bedpan during turning to prevent spillage. | [ ] | [ ] | [ ] |
| d. Wipe anal area with tissue. Wash perineum with soap and warm water. Pat dry. | [ ] | [ ] | [ ] |
| 20. Assist patient to comfortable position. | [ ] | [ ] | [ ] |
| 21. Cover bedpan and remove from bedside. Obtain specimen if required. Empty and clean bedpan and return it to bedside. | [ ] | [ ] | [ ] |
| 22. Remove and discard gloves. Wash hands. | [ ] | [ ] | [ ] |
| 23. Spray air freshener if necessary to control odor, unless contraindicated (respiratory conditions, allergies). | [ ] | [ ] | [ ] |

E = Excels;  S = Satisfactory;  U = Unsatisfactory

COMMENTS:

[ ] Pass  [ ] Fail

Student's Signature_____ Date_____

Instructor's Signature_____ Date_____

© 1992 J.B. Lippincott Company, Fundamentals of Nursing:  Human Health and Function

## PROCEDURE 28-8
## MAKING AN UNOCCUPIED BED

|  |  | E | S | U |
|---|---|---|---|---|
| 1. | Wash hands. | [ ] | [ ] | [ ] |
| 2. | Assemble equipment on bedside table or chair. | [ ] | [ ] | [ ] |
| 3. | Help patient to chair at bedside. | [ ] | [ ] | [ ] |
| 4. | Raise bed to comfortable working position. | [ ] | [ ] | [ ] |
| 5. | Loosen linen on one side of bed. Move to other side of bed and loosen all linen. | [ ] | [ ] | [ ] |
| 6. | Remove bedspread and blanket and fold each separately, if they are to be reused. Place over back of chair. | [ ] | [ ] | [ ] |
| 7. | Remove pillowcases by grasping seamed end with one hand and pulling pillow out with the other. Place pillows on chair. Discard pillowcases in linen bag. | [ ] | [ ] | [ ] |
| 8. | Remove each piece of linen separately by rolling into a ball and discarding into linen bag. Be careful to prevent soiled linen from touching your uniform. | [ ] | [ ] | [ ] |
| 9. | Slide mattress to head of bed if it has slipped to the foot. | [ ] | [ ] | [ ] |
| 10. | Wipe mattress with antiseptic solution if grossly soiled. Dry thoroughly. | [ ] | [ ] | [ ] |
| 11. | Working from side of bed where linen is stored, spread mattress pad over mattress and smooth out wrinkles. | [ ] | [ ] | [ ] |
| 12. | Unfold bottom sheet lengthwise on bed with vertical center crease along center of bed. Unfold top layer toward opposite side of mattress. Pull remaining top sheet over head of mattress, leaving bottom edge of sheet even with mattress edge. Smooth bottom sheet with hand. | [ ] | [ ] | [ ] |
| 13. | Standing near head of bed, tuck excess sheet under the mattress on your side. | [ ] | [ ] | [ ] |
| 14. | Miter the corner on you side: |  |  |  |
|  | a. Grasp side edge of sheet about 18 inches down from mattress top. | [ ] | [ ] | [ ] |
|  | b. Lay sheet on top of mattress to form triangular, flat fold. | [ ] | [ ] | [ ] |
|  | c. Tuck sheet hanging loose below mattress under the mattress, without pulling on triangular fold. | [ ] | [ ] | [ ] |
|  | d. Pick up top of triangular fold and place it over side of mattress. | [ ] | [ ] | [ ] |
|  | e. Tuck this loose portion of sheet under mattress. | [ ] | [ ] | [ ] |
| 15. | If contour sheets are used, omit Step 14 and fit elastic edges under corner of mattress. | [ ] | [ ] | [ ] |
| 16. | Tuck remaining sheet on that side under the mattress. | [ ] | [ ] | [ ] |
| 17. | Lay draw sheet, folded in half, on the bed with the center fold at center of bed. Place top edge of draw sheet about 12 to 15 inches from head of bed. Tuck excess draw sheet under mattress. | [ ] | [ ] | [ ] |

*(continued)*

© 1992 J.B. Lippincott Company, Fundamentals of Nursing: Human Health and Function

## 28-8: Making An Unoccupied Bed *(Continued)*

|  | E | S | U |
|---|---|---|---|
| 18. Move to opposite side of bed. Spread bottom sheet over mattress edge and miter top corner. | [ ] | [ ] | [ ] |
| 19. Tuck excess bottom sheet tightly under mattress, pulling gently to smooth out wrinkles. | [ ] | [ ] | [ ] |
| 20. Grasp draw sheet, pulling gently. Beginning at middle, tuck draw sheet under mattress firmly. Finish tucking top and bottom. | [ ] | [ ] | [ ] |
| 21. Return to side of bed where linen is placed. | [ ] | [ ] | [ ] |
| 22. Place top sheet on bed with vertical center fold at center of bed. Unfold sheet with seams facing out and top edge even with top of mattress. Smooth sheet, with excess falling over bottom edge of mattress. | [ ] | [ ] | [ ] |
| 23. Spread blanket and bedspread evenly over bed. | [ ] | [ ] | [ ] |
| 24. Miter the bottom corner, using all three layers of linen (sheet, blanket, bedspread). Leave sides untucked. | [ ] | [ ] | [ ] |
| 25. Move to opposite side of bed and miter bottom corner, using all three linen layers. | [ ] | [ ] | [ ] |
| 26. Standing at bottom of bed, grasp top covers about 10 inches from bottom of mattress. Loosen linen slightly by pulling on top covers or forming a pleat. | [ ] | [ ] | [ ] |
| 27. Put clean pillowcases on: | | | |
| a. Grasp center of pillowcase, with one hand on seamed end. | [ ] | [ ] | [ ] |
| b. Gather case, turning it inside out over the hand holding it. | [ ] | [ ] | [ ] |
| c. With same hand, grasp middle of one end of pillow. | [ ] | [ ] | [ ] |
| d. Pull case over pillow with free hand. | [ ] | [ ] | [ ] |
| e. Adjust case so corners fit over pillow. | [ ] | [ ] | [ ] |
| 28. Place pillows in center at head of bed. | [ ] | [ ] | [ ] |
| 29. Fold top linen back to one side or fanfold at bottom of bed. | [ ] | [ ] | [ ] |
| 30. Secure call bell within patient's reach and lower bed. | [ ] | [ ] | [ ] |
| 31. Arrange bedside table, nightstand, and personal items within easy reach. | [ ] | [ ] | [ ] |
| 32. Discard soiled linen according to agency policy. | [ ] | [ ] | [ ] |
| 33. Wash hands. | [ ] | [ ] | [ ] |

E = Excels; S = Satisfactory; U = Unsatisfactory

COMMENTS:

[ ] Pass [ ] Fail

Student's Signature_____ Date_____

Instructor's Signature_____ Date _____

© 1992 J.B. Lippincott Company, Fundamentals of Nursing: Human Health and Function

## PROCEDURE 28-9
## MAKING AN OCCUPIED BED

|  | E | S | U |
|---|---|---|---|
| 1. Wash hands. | [ ] | [ ] | [ ] |
| 2. Assemble equipment on bedside table or chair. | [ ] | [ ] | [ ] |
| 3. Close door or bedside curtains. | [ ] | [ ] | [ ] |
| 4. Lock siderail up on side of bed opposite from where clean linen is stacked. | [ ] | [ ] | [ ] |
| 5. Raise bed to comfortable working position. Lower siderail on your side of bed. | [ ] | [ ] | [ ] |
| 6. Loosen all top linen from foot of bed. | [ ] | [ ] | [ ] |
| 7. Remove bedspread and blanket separately. Without shaking, fold each and place over back of chair if they are to be reused. If they are soiled, hold them away from your uniform and place in linen bag. | [ ] | [ ] | [ ] |
| 8. Leave top sheet on patient or cover patient with a bath blanket, then remove and discard top sheet. | [ ] | [ ] | [ ] |
| 9. Loosen bottom sheet on your side. | [ ] | [ ] | [ ] |
| 10. Lower head of bed to flat position. If patient cannot tolerate flat position, lower head of bed as far as patient can tolerate. | [ ] | [ ] | [ ] |
| 11. With assistance from another worker, grasp mattress lugs and slide mattress to head of bed if it has slipped down. | [ ] | [ ] | [ ] |
| 12. Help patient roll onto side facing away from you. Have patient grasp siderail to assist. Adjust pillow under head. | [ ] | [ ] | [ ] |
| 13. Fanfold soiled draw sheet and tuck under buttocks, back, and shoulders. Repeat with soiled bottom sheet and tuck under patient. Do not fanfold mattress pad unless it is soiled. | [ ] | [ ] | [ ] |
| 14. Place clean bottom sheet on bed. Unfold lengthwise so bottom edge is even with end of mattress and vertical center crease is at center of bed. | [ ] | [ ] | [ ] |
| 15. Bring sheet's bottom edge over mattress sides and fanfold top of sheet toward center of mattress and place tightly next to patient. | [ ] | [ ] | [ ] |
| 16. Tuck top edge of sheet under mattress. Miter the corner on your side:<br>a. Grasp side edge of sheet about 18 inches down from mattress top. | [ ] | [ ] | [ ] |

*(continued)*

© 1992 J.B. Lippincott Company, Fundamentals of Nursing: Human Health and Function

28-9:  Making An Occupied Bed *(Continued)*

|  | E | S | U |
|---|---|---|---|
| b. Lay sheet on top of mattress to form triangular, flat fold. | [ ] | [ ] | [ ] |
| c. Tuck sheet hanging loose below mattress under the mattress, without pulling on triangular fold. | [ ] | [ ] | [ ] |
| d. Pick up top of triangular fold and place it over side of mattress. | [ ] | [ ] | [ ] |
| e. Tuck this loose portion of sheet under mattress. | [ ] | [ ] | [ ] |
| 17. If contour sheets are used, omit Step 14 and fit elastic edges under corner of mattress. | [ ] | [ ] | [ ] |
| 18. Tuck remaining sheet on that side under the mattress. | [ ] | [ ] | [ ] |
| 19. Place draw sheet on bed with the center fold at center of bed.  Position sheet so it will extend from patient's back to below the buttocks.  Fanfold the top edge and place next to patient.  Tuck excess under mattress. | [ ] | [ ] | [ ] |
| 20. Lock siderails up and move to opposite side of bed. | [ ] | [ ] | [ ] |
| 21. Lower siderail.  Help patient roll over folds of linen onto other side. | [ ] | [ ] | [ ] |
| 22. Move pillow under patient's head. | [ ] | [ ] | [ ]. |
| 23. Remove soiled linen by folding into a square or bundle, with soiled side turned in.  Place in linen bag. | [ ] | [ ] | [ ] |
| 24. Grasp edge of fanfolded bottom sheet.  Tuck top of sheet under top of mattress.  Miter top corner. | [ ] | [ ] | [ ] |
| 25. Facing bed, pull bottom sheet tight and tuck excess linen under mattress from top to bottom. | [ ] | [ ] | [ ] |
| 26. Unfold draw sheet by grasping at center. Tuck excess tightly under mattress.  Tuck the middle first, then top, and finally the bottom. | [ ] | [ ] | [ ] |
| 27. Help patient to center of bed. | [ ] | [ ] | [ ] |
| 28. Raise siderail if necessary and move to slide of bed where remainder of linen is stored. | [ ] | [ ] | [ ] |
| 29. Place top sheet over patient with center crease lengthwise at center of bed with seam side up.  Unfold sheet from head to toe. | [ ] | [ ] | [ ] |
| 30. Have patient grasp top edge of clean top sheet.  Remove bath blanket or soiled top linen by pulling from beneath clean top sheet.  Discard in linen bag. | [ ] | [ ] | [ ] |
| 31. Spread blanket and bedspread evenly over top of patient. | [ ] | [ ] | [ ] |
| 32. Miter the bottom corner, using all three layers of linen (sheet, blanket, bedspread).  Leave sides untucked. | [ ] | [ ] | [ ] |
| 33. Move to opposite side of bed and miter bottom corner, using all three linen layers. | [ ] | [ ] | [ ] |

*(continued)*

© 1992 J.B. Lippincott Company, Fundamentals of Nursing:  Human Health and Function

**28-9: Making An Occupied Bed** *(Continued)*

| | E | S | U |
|---|---|---|---|
| 34. Standing at bottom of bed, grasp top covers about 10 inches from bottom of mattress. Loosen linen slightly by pulling on top covers or forming a pleat. | [ ] | [ ] | [ ] |
| 35. Put clean pillowcases on: | | | |
| a. Grasp center of pillowcase, with one hand on seamed end. | [ ] | [ ] | [ ] |
| b. Gather case, turning it inside out over the hand holding it. | [ ] | [ ] | [ ] |
| c. With same hand, grasp middle of one end of pillow. | [ ] | [ ] | [ ] |
| d. Pull case over pillow with free hand. | [ ] | [ ] | [ ] |
| e. Adjust case so corners fit over pillow. | [ ] | [ ] | [ ] |
| 36. Place pillows under patient's head. | [ ] | [ ] | [ ] |
| 37. Secure call bell within patient's reach and lower bed. | [ ] | [ ] | [ ] |
| 38. Arrange bedside table, nightstand, and personal items within easy reach. | [ ] | [ ] | [ ] |
| 39. Discard soiled linen according to agency policy. | [ ] | [ ] | [ ] |
| 40. Wash hands. | [ ] | [ ] | [ ] |

E = Excels;  S = Satisfactory;  U = Unsatisfactory

COMMENTS:

[ ] Pass  [ ] Fail

Student's Signature_____ Date_____

Instructor's Signature_____ Date_____

© 1992 J.B. Lippincott Company, Fundamentals of Nursing:  Human Health and Function

## PROCEDURE 29-1
## USING PROPER BODY MECHANICS

|  | E | S | U |
|---|---|---|---|
| 1. Wash hands. | [ ] | [ ] | [ ] |
| 2. Plan movement before doing it: | | | |
|    a. Lock wheels on bed, stretcher, or wheelchair. | [ ] | [ ] | [ ] |
|    b. Allow patient to assist during transfer. | [ ] | [ ] | [ ] |
|    c. Use mechanical aids or additional personnel to move heavy patients. | [ ] | [ ] | [ ] |
|    d. Slide, push, or pull patient rather than lifting and carrying when possible. | [ ] | [ ] | [ ] |
|    e. Tighten abdominal and gluteal muscles before lifting or moving patient. | [ ] | [ ] | [ ] |
|    f. Use smooth, rhythmic, coordinated movements. | [ ] | [ ] | [ ] |
|    g. Plan movements before beginning when another person is assisting. | [ ] | [ ] | [ ] |
| 3. Begin all movements with proper body alignment and balance: | | | |
|    a. Face patient to be lifted and pivot your body. | [ ] | [ ] | [ ] |
|    b. Increase base of support by placing both feet flat on floor, knees slightly bent, with one foot slightly in front of the other or one step apart. | [ ] | [ ] | [ ] |
|    c. Lower center of gravity toward patient to be transferred. | [ ] | [ ] | [ ] |
| 4. Elevate adjustable beds to waist level and lower siderails to prevent stretching. | [ ] | [ ] | [ ] |
| 5. Carry objects close to body and stand as close as possible to work area. | [ ] | [ ] | [ ] |

E = Excels;  S = Satisfactory;  U = Unsatisfactory

COMMENTS:

[ ] Pass  [ ] Fail

Student's Signature_____ Date_____

Instructor's Signature_____ Date _____

© 1992 J.B. Lippincott Company, Fundamentals of Nursing: Human Health and Function

# PROCEDURE 29-2A
## POSITIONING A PATIENT IN BED
### MOVING A PATIENT UP IN BED
#### (One Nurse)

|  | E | S | U |
|---|---|---|---|
| 1. Wash hands. | [ ] | [ ] | [ ] |
| 2. Explain procedure and rationale to patient. | [ ] | [ ] | [ ] |
| 3. Lower head of bed to flat position and raise level of bed to comfortable working height. | [ ] | [ ] | [ ] |
| 4. Remove all pillows from under patient. Leave one at head of bed. | [ ] | [ ] | [ ] |
| 5. Instruct patient to bend legs, put feet flat on bed, and place arm nearest you under your arm and around your shoulder. | [ ] | [ ] | [ ] |
| 6. Place your feet in broad stance with one foot in front of the other. Flex your knees and thighs. | [ ] | [ ] | [ ] |
| 7. Place one arm under patient's shoulders and one arm under thighs. | [ ] | [ ] | [ ] |
| 8. Rock back and forth on front and back leg to count of three. On third count, patient pushes with feet as you lift and pull patient up in bed. | [ ] | [ ] | [ ] |
| 9. Elevate head of bed and place pillows under head. Raise siderails and lower bed to lowest level. | [ ] | [ ] | [ ] |

E = Excels;  S = Satisfactory;  U = Unsatisfactory

COMMENTS:

[ ] Pass  [ ] Fail

Student's Signature_____ Date_____

Instructor's Signature_____ Date_____

© 1992 J.B. Lippincott Company, Fundamentals of Nursing: Human Health and Function

# PROCEDURE 29-2B
# POSITIONING A PATIENT IN BED
## MOVING HELPLESS PATIENT UP IN BED
### (Two Nurses)

|  |  | E | S | U |
|---|---|---|---|---|
| 1. | Wash hands. | [ ] | [ ] | [ ] |
| 2. | Explain procedure and rationale to patient. | [ ] | [ ] | [ ] |
| 3. | Lower head of bed to flat position and raise level of bed to comfortable working height. | [ ] | [ ] | [ ] |
| 4. | Remove all pillows from under patient. Leave one at head of bed. | [ ] | [ ] | [ ] |
| 5. | One nurse stands on each side of bed with wide base of support and one foot slightly in front of the other. | [ ] | [ ] | [ ] |
| 6. | Each nurse rolls up and grasps edges of turn sheet close to patient's shoulders and buttocks. | [ ] | [ ] | [ ] |
| 7. | Flex knees and hips. Tighten abdominal and gluteal muscles. | [ ] | [ ] | [ ] |
| 8. | Rock back and forth on front and back leg to count of three. On third count, both nurses shift weight to front leg as they simultaneously lift patient toward head of bed. | [ ] | [ ] | [ ] |
| 9. | Elevate head of bed and place pillows under patient's head. Adjust other positioning pillows as necessary. Put up siderails and lower bed to lowest level. | [ ] | [ ] | [ ] |

E = Excels;  S = Satisfactory;  U = Unsatisfactory

COMMENTS:

[ ] Pass  [ ] Fail

Student's Signature_____ Date_____

Instructor's Signature_____ Date _____

© 1992 J.B. Lippincott Company, Fundamentals of Nursing: Human Health and Function

# PROCEDURE 29-2C
## POSITIONING A PATIENT IN BED
### POSITIONING PATIENT IN SIDE-LYING POSITION

|  | E | S | U |
|---|---|---|---|
| 1. Wash hands. | [ ] | [ ] | [ ] |
| 2. Lower head of bed as flat as patient can tolerate. | [ ] | [ ] | [ ] |
| 3. Elevate and lock siderail on side patient will face when turned. | [ ] | [ ] | [ ] |
| 4. Place arm that patient will turn toward away from his or her body. Fold other arm across chest. | [ ] | [ ] | [ ] |
| 5. Flex patient's knee that will not be next to mattress after turn. | [ ] | [ ] | [ ] |
| 6. Go around to other side of bed. Assume a broad stance with knees slightly flexed. | [ ] | [ ] | [ ] |
| 7. Place one hand on patient's hip and one hand on his or her far shoulder. | [ ] | [ ] | [ ] |
| 8. Roll patient toward you. | [ ] | [ ] | [ ] |
| 9. Align patient properly and place pillow under head. | [ ] | [ ] | [ ] |
| 10. Pull shoulder blade forward and out from under patient. Support upper arm with pillow. | [ ] | [ ] | [ ] |
| 11. Fold a pillow lengthwise or roll a towel or bath blanket and tuck behind patient's back. | [ ] | [ ] | [ ] |
| 12. Place pillow lengthwise between patient's legs from thighs to feet. | [ ] | [ ] | [ ] |

E = Excels;  S = Satisfactory;  U = Unsatisfactory

COMMENTS:

[ ] Pass  [ ] Fail

Student's Signature_____ Date_____

Instructor's Signature_____ Date_____

© 1992 J.B. Lippincott Company, Fundamentals of Nursing: Human Health and Function

## PROCEDURE 29-2D
## POSITIONING A PATIENT IN BED
## LOGROLLING

|  | E | S | U |
|---|---|---|---|
| 1. Wash hands. | [ ] | [ ] | [ ] |
| 2. Obtain assistance of two or three other nurses. | [ ] | [ ] | [ ] |
| 3. All nurses stand on same side of bed, with feet apart, one foot slightly ahead of the other. Flex knees and hips. | [ ] | [ ] | [ ] |
| 4. Place one pillow to support head during and after turn. | [ ] | [ ] | [ ] |
| 5. Place pillows between patient's legs. | [ ] | [ ] | [ ] |
| 6. Reach across patient and support head, thorax, trunk, and legs. | [ ] | [ ] | [ ] |
| 7. On count of three, roll patient in one coordinated movement to lateral position. | [ ] | [ ] | [ ] |
| 8. Align patient properly and place pillow under head. | [ ] | [ ] | [ ] |
| 9. Support upper arm with pillow. | [ ] | [ ] | [ ] |
| 10. Fold pillow lengthwise or roll a towel or bath blanket and tuck behind patient's back. | [ ] | [ ] | [ ] |
| 11. Place pillow lengthwise between patient's legs from thighs to feet. | [ ] | [ ] | [ ] |

E = Excels;  S = Satisfactory;  U = Unsatisfactory

COMMENTS:

[ ] Pass  [ ] Fail

Student's Signature_____ Date_____

Instructor's Signature_____ Date_____

© 1992 J.B. Lippincott Company, Fundamentals of Nursing:  Human Health and Function

## PROCEDURE 29-3
## PROVIDING RANGE-OF-MOTION EXERCISES

|  |  | E | S | U |
|---|---|---|---|---|
| 1. | Wash hands. | [ ] | [ ] | [ ] |
| 2. | Explain procedure and rationale to patient. | [ ] | [ ] | [ ] |
| 3. | Position patient on back with head of bed as flat as possible. Elevate bed to comfortable working height. | [ ] | [ ] | [ ] |
| 4. | Stand on side of bed of joints to be exercised. Uncover limb to be exercised only. | [ ] | [ ] | [ ] |
| 5. | Perform exercises slowly and gently, providing support by holding areas proximal and distal to the joint. | [ ] | [ ] | [ ] |
| 6. | Repeat exercises to each joint five times. | [ ] | [ ] | [ ] |
| 7. | Discontinue or decrease ROM if patient complains of discomfort or muscle spasm. | [ ] | [ ] | [ ] |
| 8. | Neck: | | | |
| | a. Bring chin to chest. | [ ] | [ ] | [ ] |
| | b. Bend head toward back. | [ ] | [ ] | [ ] |
| | c. Tilt head toward each shoulder. | [ ] | [ ] | [ ] |
| | d. Rotate head in circular motion. | [ ] | [ ] | [ ] |
| | e. Return to erect position. | [ ] | [ ] | [ ] |
| 9. | Shoulder: | | | |
| | a. Raise arm from side to above head. | [ ] | [ ] | [ ] |
| | b. Abduct and rotate shoulder by raising arm above head with palm up. | [ ] | [ ] | [ ] |
| | c. Adduct shoulder by moving arm across body as far as possible. | [ ] | [ ] | [ ] |
| | d. Rotate shoulder internally and externally by flexing elbow and moving forearm to touch palm on mattress, then up until back of hand touches mattress. | [ ] | [ ] | [ ] |
| | e. Move shoulder in a full circle. | [ ] | [ ] | [ ] |
| 10. | Elbow: | | | |
| | a. Bend elbow toward shoulder. | [ ] | [ ] | [ ] |
| | b. Hyperextend elbow as far as possible. | [ ] | [ ] | [ ] |
| 11. | Wrist and hand: | | | |
| | a. Move hand toward inner aspect of forearm. | [ ] | [ ] | [ ] |
| | b. Bend dorsal surface of hand backward. | [ ] | [ ] | [ ] |
| | c. Abduct wrist by bending toward thumb. | [ ] | [ ] | [ ] |
| | d. Adduct wrist by bending toward fifth finger. | [ ] | [ ] | [ ] |
| | e. Make a fist, then extend the fingers. | [ ] | [ ] | [ ] |
| | f. Spread fingers apart, then bring together. | [ ] | [ ] | [ ] |
| | g. Move thumb across hand to base of fifth finger. | [ ] | [ ] | [ ] |
| 12. | Hip and knee: | | | |
| | a. Lift leg and bend knee toward chest. | [ ] | [ ] | [ ] |

*(continued)*

© 1992 J.B. Lippincott Company, Fundamentals of Nursing: Human Health and Function

## 29-3:  Providing Range-of-Motion Exercises *(Continued)*

|  | E | S | U |
|---|---|---|---|
| b. Abduct and adduct leg, moving leg laterally away from body and returning to medial position. | [ ] | [ ] | [ ] |
| c. Internally and externally rotate hip by turning leg inward then outward. | [ ] | [ ] | [ ] |
| d. Take special care to support joints of larger limbs. | [ ] | [ ] | [ ] |
| 13.  Ankle and foot: | | | |
| a. Dorsiflex foot by moving foot so toes point upward. | [ ] | [ ] | [ ] |
| b. Plantarflex by moving foot so toes point downward. | [ ] | [ ] | [ ] |
| c. Curl toes down, then extend. | [ ] | [ ] | [ ] |
| d. Spread toes apart, then bring together. | [ ] | [ ] | [ ] |
| e. Invert by turning sole of foot medially. | [ ] | [ ] | [ ] |
| f. Evert by turning sole of foot laterally. | [ ] | [ ] | [ ] |
| 14.  Move to other side of bed and repeat exercises. | [ ] | [ ] | [ ] |
| 15.  Reposition patient to position of comfort. | [ ] | [ ] | [ ] |
| 16.  Document ROM. | [ ] | [ ] | [ ] |

E = Excels;  S = Satisfactory;  U = Unsatisfactory

COMMENTS:

[ ] Pass  [ ] Fail

Student's Signature_____  Date_____

Instructor's Signature_____  Date _____

© 1992 J.B. Lippincott Company, Fundamentals of Nursing:  Human Health and Function

# PROCEDURE 29-4A
## ASSISTING WITH AMBULATION
### ONE NURSE

|  | E | S | U |
|---|---|---|---|
| 1. Wash hands. | [ ] | [ ] | [ ] |
| 2. Explain procedure and rationale for ambulation to patient. Decide together how far and where to ambulate. | [ ] | [ ] | [ ] |
| 3. Place bed in lowest position. | [ ] | [ ] | [ ] |
| 4. Assist patient to sitting position on side of bed. Assess for dizziness or faintness. Obtain orthostatic vital signs if complaints are present. Allow patient to remain in this position until he or she feels secure. | [ ] | [ ] | [ ] |
| 5. Help patient don robe and footwear. | [ ] | [ ] | [ ] |
| 6. Wrap transfer belt around patient's waist (optional according to assessment). | [ ] | [ ] | [ ] |
| 7. Assist patient to standing position and assess patient's balance. Return to bed or transfer to chair if very weak or unsteady. | [ ] | [ ] | [ ] |
| 8. Position yourself behind patient while supporting him or her by waist or transfer belt. | [ ] | [ ] | [ ] |
| 9. Take several steps forward with patient, assessing strength and balance. | [ ] | [ ] | [ ] |
| 10. If patient has one-sided weakness, stand on the affected side and provide support by placing arm nearest patient around his or her waist. Place other hand around patient's upper arm on affected side. | [ ] | [ ] | [ ] |
| 11. Encourage patient to use good posture and to look ahead, not down at feet. | [ ] | [ ] | [ ] |
| 12. Ambulate for planned distance or time. | [ ] | [ ] | [ ] |
| 13. If patient becomes weak or dizzy, return to bed or assist to chair. | [ ] | [ ] | [ ] |
| 14. If patient begins to fall, place your feet wide apart with one foot in front. Support patient by pulling his or her weight backward against your body. Lower gently to floor, protecting head. | [ ] | [ ] | [ ] |

E = Excels;  S = Satisfactory;  U = Unsatisfactory

COMMENTS:

[ ] Pass  [ ] Fail

Student's Signature_____ Date_____

Instructor's Signature_____ Date _____

© 1992 J.B. Lippincott Company, Fundamentals of Nursing:  Human Health and Function

## PROCEDURE 29-4B
## ASSISTING WITH AMBULATION
### TWO NURSES

|  | E | S | U |
|---|---|---|---|
| 1. Wash hands. | [ ] | [ ] | [ ] |
| 2. Explain procedure and rationale for ambulation to patient. Decide together how far and where to ambulate. | [ ] | [ ] | [ ] |
| 3. Place bed in lowest position. | [ ] | [ ] | [ ] |
| 4. Assist patient to sitting position on side of bed. Assess for dizziness or faintness. Obtain orthostatic vital signs if complaints are present. Allow patient to remain in this position until he or she feels secure. | [ ] | [ ] | [ ] |
| 5. Help patient don robe and footwear. | [ ] | [ ] | [ ] |
| 6. Wrap transfer belt around patient's waist. (Optional according to assessment.) | [ ] | [ ] | [ ] |
| 7. Assist patient to standing position with one nurse on each side. | [ ] | [ ] | [ ] |
| 8. Each nurse grasps patient's upper arm with the nearest hand and the elbow with the other hand. | [ ] | [ ] | [ ] |
| 9. If transfer belt is used, each nurse grasps belt with near hand and elbow with other hand. | [ ] | [ ] | [ ] |
| 10. Walk with patient using slow, even steps. Assess strength and balance. | [ ] | [ ] | [ ] |
| 11. Encourage patient to use good posture and to look ahead, not down at feet. | [ ] | [ ] | [ ] |
| 12. If patient becomes weak or dizzy, return to bed or assist to chair. | [ ] | [ ] | [ ] |
| 13. If patient begins to fall, lower gently to floor. | [ ] | [ ] | [ ] |

E = Excels;  S = Satisfactory;  U = Unsatisfactory

COMMENTS:

[ ] Pass  [ ] Fail

Student's Signature_____ Date_____

Instructor's Signature_____ Date_____

© 1992 J.B. Lippincott Company, Fundamentals of Nursing: Human Health and Function

# PROCEDURE 29-4C
# ASSISTING WITH AMBULATION
## USING A WALKER

| | E | S | U |
|---|---|---|---|
| 1. Wash hands. | [ ] | [ ] | [ ] |
| 2. Explain procedure and rationale for ambulation to patient. Decide together how far and where to ambulate. | [ ] | [ ] | [ ] |
| 3. Place bed in lowest position. | [ ] | [ ] | [ ] |
| 4. Assist patient to sitting position on side of bed. Assess for dizziness or faintness. Obtain orthostatic vital signs if complaints are present. Allow patient to remain in this position until he or she feels secure. | [ ] | [ ] | [ ] |
| 5. Help patient don robe and footwear. | [ ] | [ ] | [ ] |
| 6. Assist patient to standing position. | [ ] | [ ] | [ ] |
| 7. Have patient grasp walker handles. | [ ] | [ ] | [ ] |
| 8. Patient moves walker ahead 6 to 8 inches, placing all four feet of walker on floor. | [ ] | [ ] | [ ] |
| 9. Patient moves forward to walker. | [ ] | [ ] | [ ] |
| 10. Nurse walks closely behind and slightly to side of patient. | [ ] | [ ] | [ ] |
| 11. Repeat above sequence until walk is complete. | [ ] | [ ] | [ ] |
| 12. If patient becomes weak or dizzy, return to bed or assist to chair. | [ ] | [ ] | [ ] |
| 13. If patient begins to fall, lower gently to floor. | [ ] | [ ] | [ ] |

E = Excels;  S = Satisfactory;  U = Unsatisfactory

COMMENTS:

[ ] Pass  [ ] Fail

Student's Signature_____ Date_____

Instructor's Signature_____ Date_____

© 1992 J.B. Lippincott Company, Fundamentals of Nursing: Human Health and Function

66

## PROCEDURE 29-5A
# HELPING PATIENTS WITH CRUTCH WALKING
## FOUR-POINT GAIT

|  | E | S | U |
|---|---|---|---|
| 1. Wash hands. | [ ] | [ ] | [ ] |
| 2. Instruct patient to stand erect, facing forward in tripod position, placing crutch tips 6 inches in front of feet and 6 inches to side of each foot. | [ ] | [ ] | [ ] |
| 3. Patient moves right crutch forward 4 to 6 inches. | [ ] | [ ] | [ ] |
| 4. Patient moves left foot forward to level of right crutch. | [ ] | [ ] | [ ] |
| 5. Patient moves left crutch forward 4 to 6 inches. | [ ] | [ ] | [ ] |
| 6. Patient moves right foot forward to level of left crutch. | [ ] | [ ] | [ ] |
| 7. Repeat sequence. | [ ] | [ ] | [ ] |

E = Excels;  S = Satisfactory;  U = Unsatisfactory

COMMENTS:

[ ] Pass  [ ] Fail

Student's Signature_____ Date_____

Instructor's Signature_____ Date _____

© 1992 J.B. Lippincott Company, Fundamentals of Nursing: Human Health and Function

**PROCEDURE 29-5B**
# HELPING PATIENTS WITH CRUTCH WALKING
## THREE-POINT GAIT

|  | E | S | U |
|---|---|---|---|
| 1. Wash hands. | [ ] | [ ] | [ ] |
| 2. Instruct patient to stand erect, facing forward in tripod position, placing crutch tips 6 inches in front of feet and 6 inches to side of each foot. | [ ] | [ ] | [ ] |
| 3. Patient moves both crutches and affected leg forward. | [ ] | [ ] | [ ] |
| 4. Patient moves stronger leg forward, bearing entire weight on stronger leg. | [ ] | [ ] | [ ] |
| 5. Repeat sequence. | [ ] | [ ] | [ ] |

E = Excels;  S = Satisfactory;  U = Unsatisfactory

COMMENTS:

[ ] Pass  [ ] Fail

Student's Signature_____ Date_____

Instructor's Signature_____ Date _____

© 1992 J.B. Lippincott Company, Fundamentals of Nursing:  Human Health and Function

## PROCEDURE 29-5C
# HELPING PATIENTS WITH CRUTCH WALKING
## TWO-POINT GAIT

|  | E | S | U |
|---|---|---|---|
| 1. Wash hands. | [ ] | [ ] | [ ] |
| 2. Instruct patient to stand erect, facing forward in tripod position, placing crutch tips 6 inches in front of feet and 6 inches to side of each foot. | [ ] | [ ] | [ ] |
| 3. Patient moves left crutch and right foot forward. | [ ] | [ ] | [ ] |
| 4. Patient moves right crutch and left foot forward. | [ ] | [ ] | [ ] |
| 5. Repeat sequence. | [ ] | [ ] | [ ] |

E = Excels;  S = Satisfactory;  U = Unsatisfactory

COMMENTS:

[ ] Pass  [ ] Fail

Student's Signature_____ Date_____

Instructor's Signature_____ Date _____

© 1992 J.B. Lippincott Company, Fundamentals of Nursing:  Human Health and Function

# PROCEDURE 29-5D
# HELPING PATIENTS WITH CRUTCH WALKING
## SWINGING-TO GAIT

|  |  | E | S | U |
|---|---|---|---|---|
| 1. | Wash hands. | [ ] | [ ] | [ ] |
| 2. | Instruct patient to stand erect, facing forward in tripod position, placing crutch tips 6 inches in front of feet and 6 inches to side of each foot. | [ ] | [ ] | [ ] |
| 3. | Patient moves both crutches forward. | [ ] | [ ] | [ ] |
| 4. | Patient lifts legs and swings to crutches, supporting body weight on crutches. | [ ] | [ ] | [ ] |
| 5. | Repeat sequence. | [ ] | [ ] | [ ] |

E = Excels;  S = Satisfactory;  U = Unsatisfactory

COMMENTS:

[ ] Pass  [ ] Fail

Student's Signature_____ Date_____

Instructor's Signature_____ Date_____

© 1992 J.B. Lippincott Company, Fundamentals of Nursing: Human Health and Function

## PROCEDURE 29-5E
# HELPING PATIENTS WITH CRUTCH WALKING
## SWINGING-THROUGH GAIT

|  | | E | S | U |
|---|---|---|---|---|
| 1. | Wash hands. | [ ] | [ ] | [ ] |
| 2. | Instruct patient to stand erect, facing forward in tripod position, placing crutch tips 6 inches in front of feet and 6 inches to side of each foot. | [ ] | [ ] | [ ] |
| 3. | Patient moves both crutches forward. | [ ] | [ ] | [ ] |
| 4. | Patient lifts legs and swings through and ahead of crutches, supporting weight on crutches. | [ ] | [ ] | [ ] |
| 5. | Repeat sequence. | [ ] | [ ] | [ ] |

E = Excels;  S = Satisfactory;  U = Unsatisfactory

COMMENTS:

[ ] Pass  [ ] Fail

Student's Signature_____ Date_____

Instructor's Signature_____ Date _____

© 1992 J.B. Lippincott Company, Fundamentals of Nursing:  Human Health and Function

**PROCEDURE 29-5F**
# HELPING PATIENTS WITH CRUTCH WALKING
## CLIMBING STAIRS

|  |  | E | S | U |
|---|---|---|---|---|
| 1. | Wash hands. | [ ] | [ ] | [ ] |
| 2. | Instruct patient to stand erect, facing stairs in tripod position, placing crutch tips 6 inches in front of feet and 6 inches to side of each foot. | [ ] | [ ] | [ ] |
| 3. | Patient transfers body weight to crutches. | [ ] | [ ] | [ ] |
| 4. | Patient places unaffected leg on step. | [ ] | [ ] | [ ] |
| 5. | Patient transfers body weight to unaffected leg. | [ ] | [ ] | [ ] |
| 6. | Patient moves crutches and affected leg to step. | [ ] | [ ] | [ ] |
| 7. | Repeat sequence to top of stairs. | [ ] | [ ] | [ ] |

E = Excels;  S = Satisfactory;  U = Unsatisfactory

COMMENTS:

[ ] Pass  [ ] Fail

Student's Signature_____ Date_____

Instructor's Signature_____ Date _____

© 1992 J.B. Lippincott Company, Fundamentals of Nursing:  Human Health and Function

**PROCEDURE 29-5G**
# HELPING PATIENTS WITH CRUTCH WALKING
## DESCENDING STAIRS

|  | E | S | U |
|---|---|---|---|
| 1. Wash hands. | [ ] | [ ] | [ ] |
| 2. Instruct patient to stand erect, facing stairs in tripod position. | [ ] | [ ] | [ ] |
| 3. Patient transfers body weight to unaffected leg. | [ ] | [ ] | [ ] |
| 4. Patient places crutches onto step and moves affected leg down to stair. | [ ] | [ ] | [ ] |
| 5. Patient transfers body weight to crutches. | [ ] | [ ] | [ ] |
| 6. Patient moves unaffected leg to stair. | [ ] | [ ] | [ ] |
| 7. Repeat sequence to bottom of stairs. | [ ] | [ ] | [ ] |

E = Excels;  S = Satisfactory;  U = Unsatisfactory

COMMENTS:

[ ] Pass  [ ] Fail

Student's Signature_____ Date_____

Instructor's Signature_____ Date _____

© 1992 J.B. Lippincott Company, Fundamentals of Nursing:  Human Health and Function

# PROCEDURE 29-6
## TRANSFERRING A PATIENT TO A STRETCHER

|  | E | S | U |
|---|---|---|---|
| 1. Wash hands. | [ ] | [ ] | [ ] |
| 2. Explain procedure and rationale to patient. | [ ] | [ ] | [ ] |
| 3. Place stretcher parallel to bed. | [ ] | [ ] | [ ] |
| 4. Raise bed to same level as stretcher. Lower siderails. Lock wheels on bed. | [ ] | [ ] | [ ] |
| 5. One or two nurses stand on side of bed without stretcher. Two nurses stand on side of bed with stretcher. | [ ] | [ ] | [ ] |
| 6. Loosen draw sheet on both sides of bed. | [ ] | [ ] | [ ] |
| 7. Nurses on side without stretcher help patient to roll toward them onto his or her side, using draw sheet to pull patient onto side or using logrolling technique. | [ ] | [ ] | [ ] |
| 8. Nurses on stretcher side of bed, slide sled board under draw sheet and under patient's buttocks and back. | [ ] | [ ] | [ ] |
| 9. Roll patient onto sled board into supine position. Place patient's arms across chest. | [ ] | [ ] | [ ] |
| 10. Move stretcher parallel to bed and lock wheels. | [ ] | [ ] | [ ] |
| 11. Nurses on stretcher side of bed assume a broad stance. | [ ] | [ ] | [ ] |
| 12. Wrap end of draw sheet over curved end of sled board and slide patient onto stretcher on count of three. | [ ] | [ ] | [ ] |
| 13. Lock siderails up on bed side of stretcher and move stretcher away from bed. | [ ] | [ ] | [ ] |
| 14. Roll patient slightly up onto side and pull sled board out from under him or her. | [ ] | [ ] | [ ] |
| 15. Lock other siderails up on stretcher. | [ ] | [ ] | [ ] |
| 16. Place cover over patient and lock safety belts across patient's chest and waist. Adjust head of stretcher according to patient limitations. | [ ] | [ ] | [ ] |

E = Excels;  S = Satisfactory;  U = Unsatisfactory

COMMENTS:

[ ] Pass  [ ] Fail

Student's Signature_____ Date_____

Instructor's Signature_____ Date_____

© 1992 J.B. Lippincott Company, Fundamentals of Nursing: Human Health and Function

## PROCEDURE 29-7
## TRANSFERRING A PATIENT TO A WHEELCHAIR

|  | | E | S | U |
|---|---|---|---|---|
| 1. | Wash hands. | [ ] | [ ] | [ ] |
| 2. | Explain procedure to patient. | [ ] | [ ] | [ ] |
| 3. | Position wheelchair at 45° angle or parallel to bed. Remove footrests and lock brakes. | [ ] | [ ] | [ ] |
| 4. | Assist patient to side-lying position, facing the side of bed he or she will sit on. | [ ] | [ ] | [ ] |
| 5. | Lock bed brakes; lower bed to lowest level and raise head of bed as far as patient can tolerate. | [ ] | [ ] | [ ] |
| 6. | Lower siderail and stand near patient's hips with foot near head of bed in front of and apart from other foot. | [ ] | [ ] | [ ] |
| 7. | Place one arm under patient's shoulders and one arm over patient's thighs. | [ ] | [ ] | [ ] |
| 8. | Swing patient's legs over side of bed. At the same time, pivot on your back leg to lift patient's trunk and shoulders. | [ ] | [ ] | [ ] |
| 9. | Stand in front of patient and assess for balance and dizziness. | [ ] | [ ] | [ ] |
| 10. | Help patient to don robe and nonskid footwear. | [ ] | [ ] | [ ] |
| 11. | Apply transfer belt if necessary. | [ ] | [ ] | [ ] |
| 12. | Spread your feet apart and flex your hips and knees. | [ ] | [ ] | [ ] |
| 13. | Put your hands around patient's waist or grasp back of transfer belt. | [ ] | [ ] | [ ] |
| 14. | Have patient slide buttocks to edge of bed until feet touch floor. | [ ] | [ ] | [ ] |
| 15. | Rock back and forth until patient stands on a count of three. | [ ] | [ ] | [ ] |
| 16. | Brace your front knee against patient's weak knee as patient stands. | [ ] | [ ] | [ ] |
| 17. | Pivot on back foot until patient feels wheelchair against back of legs, keeping your knee against the patient's knee. | [ ] | [ ] | [ ] |
| 18. | Instruct patient to place hands on chair armrests for support. Flex your knees and hips as you assist patient into chair. | [ ] | [ ] | [ ] |
| 19. | Assess patient's alignment in chair, and secure with restraints as necessary. | [ ] | [ ] | [ ] |

E = Excels;  S = Satisfactory;  U = Unsatisfactory

COMMENTS:


[ ] Pass  [ ] Fail

Student's Signature_____ Date_____

Instructor's Signature_____ Date _____

© 1992 J.B. Lippincott Company, Fundamentals of Nursing:  Human Health and Function

# PROCEDURE 30-1A
# TEACHING DEEP-BREATHING EXERCISES

|  |  | E | S | U |
|---|---|---|---|---|
| 1. | Assist patient to Fowler's or sitting position. | [ ] | [ ] | [ ] |
| 2. | Have patient place hands palm down, with middle fingers touching, along lower border of rib cage. | [ ] | [ ] | [ ] |
| 3. | Ask patient to inhale slowly through the nose, feeling middle fingers separate. Hold breath for 2 or 3 seconds. | [ ] | [ ] | [ ] |
| 4. | Have patient exhale slowly through mouth. Repeat 3 to 5 times. | [ ] | [ ] | [ ] |

E = Excels;  S = Satisfactory;  U = Unsatisfactory

COMMENTS:

[ ] Pass  [ ] Fail

Student's Signature_____ Date_____

Instructor's Signature_____ Date_____

© 1992 J.B. Lippincott Company, Fundamentals of Nursing: Human Health and Function

## PROCEDURE 30-1B
## TEACHING COUGHING AND DEEP-BREATHING EXERCISES

|  | E | S | U |
|---|---|---|---|
| 1. Assist patient to Fowler's or sitting position. | [ ] | [ ] | [ ] |

**Deep-Breathing**

|  | E | S | U |
|---|---|---|---|
| 2. Have patient place hands palm down, with middle fingers touching, along lower border of rib cage. | [ ] | [ ] | [ ] |
| 3. Ask patient to inhale slowly through the nose, feeling middle fingers separate. Hold breath for 2 or 3 seconds. | [ ] | [ ] | [ ] |
| 4. Have patient exhale slowly through mouth. Repeat 3 to 5 times. | [ ] | [ ] | [ ] |

**Controlled Coughing**

|  | E | S | U |
|---|---|---|---|
| 5. If voluntary coughing does not occur, have patient take a deep breath, hold for 3 seconds and cough deeply 2 or 3 times. Nurse stands to the patient's side to ensure the cough is not directed at him or her. | [ ] | [ ] | [ ] |
| 6. If patient has an abdominal or chest incision that will be painful during coughing, instruct patient to hold a pillow firmly over the incision (splinting) when coughing. | [ ] | [ ] | [ ] |
| 7. Instruct, reinforce, and supervise deep-breathing and coughing exercises every 2 to 3 hours post-operatively. | [ ] | [ ] | [ ] |
| 8. Document procedure. | [ ] | [ ] | [ ] |

E = Excels;  S = Satisfactory;  U = Unsatisfactory

COMMENTS:

[ ] Pass  [ ] Fail

Student's Signature_____ Date_____

Instructor's Signature_____ Date _____

© 1992 J.B. Lippincott Company, Fundamentals of Nursing: Human Health and Function

## PROCEDURE 30-2
# PROMOTING BREATHING WITH THE INCENTIVE SPIROMETER

|  |  | E | S | U |
|---|---|---|---|---|
| 1. | Wash hands. | [ ] | [ ] | [ ] |
| 2. | Assist patient to high Fowler's or sitting position. | [ ] | [ ] | [ ] |
| 3. | Instruct patient in procedure: | | | |
|  | a. Seal lips tightly around mouthpiece. | [ ] | [ ] | [ ] |
|  | b. Inhale slowly and deeply through mouth. Hold breath for 2 or 3 seconds. | [ ] | [ ] | [ ] |
|  | c. Exhale slowly around mouthpiece. | [ ] | [ ] | [ ] |
|  | d. Breathe normally for several breaths. | [ ] | [ ] | [ ] |
| 4. | Repeat procedure 5 to 10 times every 1 to 2 hours, per physician's orders. | [ ] | [ ] | [ ] |
| 5. | Wash hands. | [ ] | [ ] | [ ] |

E = Excels;  S = Satisfactory;  U = Unsatisfactory

COMMENTS:

[ ] Pass  [ ] Fail

Student's Signature_____ Date_____

Instructor's Signature_____ Date _____

© 1992 J.B. Lippincott Company, Fundamentals of Nursing: Human Health and Function

## PROCEDURE 30-3A
# ADMINISTERING OXYGEN BY NASAL CANNULA

|  | E | S | U |
|---|---|---|---|
| 1. Wash hands. | [ ] | [ ] | [ ] |
| 2. Explain procedure to patient. Encourage patient to breathe through nose. | [ ] | [ ] | [ ] |
| 3. Assist patient to semi- or high-Fowler's position, if tolerated. | [ ] | [ ] | [ ] |
| 4. Attach humidifier flow meter. Attach oxygen to humidifier nozzle, particularly if using a high oxygen flow. | [ ] | [ ] | [ ] |
| 5. Turn on the oxygen at the prescribed rate. Check that oxygen is flowing through tubing. | [ ] | [ ] | [ ] |
| 6. Place cannula prongs into nares. | [ ] | [ ] | [ ] |
| 7. Wrap tubing over and behind ears. | [ ] | [ ] | [ ] |
| 8. Adjust plastic slide under chin until cannula fits snugly. | [ ] | [ ] | [ ] |
| 9. Assess for proper functioning of equipment and observe patient's initial response to therapy. | [ ] | [ ] | [ ] |
| 10. Monitor continuous therapy by assessing for pressure areas on the skin and nares every 2 hours and rechecking flow rate every 4 to 8 hours. | [ ] | [ ] | [ ] |
| 11. Document procedure and observations. | [ ] | [ ] | [ ] |

E = Excels;  S = Satisfactory;  U = Unsatisfactory

COMMENTS:

[ ] Pass  [ ] Fail

Student's Signature_____  Date_____

Instructor's Signature_____  Date _____

© 1992 J.B. Lippincott Company, Fundamentals of Nursing: Human Health and Function

# PROCEDURE 30-3B
## ADMINISTERING OXYGEN BY MASK

| | E | S | U |
|---|---|---|---|
| 1. Wash hands. | [ ] | [ ] | [ ] |
| 2. Explain procedure to patient. | [ ] | [ ] | [ ] |
| 3. Assist patient to semi- or high-Fowler's position, if tolerated. | [ ] | [ ] | [ ] |
| 4. Attach humidifier flow meter. Attach oxygen to humidifier nozzle, particularly if using a high oxygen flow. | [ ] | [ ] | [ ] |
| 5. Turn on the oxygen at the prescribed rate. Check that oxygen is flowing through tubing. | [ ] | [ ] | [ ] |
| 6. Place mask on face, applying from the nose and over the chin. | [ ] | [ ] | [ ] |
| 7. Adjust metal rim over the nose and contour the mask to the face. | [ ] | [ ] | [ ] |
| 8. Adjust elastic band around head so mask fits snugly. | [ ] | [ ] | [ ] |
| 9. Assess for proper functioning of equipment and observe patient's initial response to therapy. | [ ] | [ ] | [ ] |
| 10. Monitor continuous therapy by assessing for pressure areas on the skin and nares every 2 hours and rechecking flow rate every 4 to 8 hours. | [ ] | [ ] | [ ] |
| 11. Document procedure and observations. | [ ] | [ ] | [ ] |

E = Excels;  S = Satisfactory;  U = Unsatisfactory

COMMENTS:

[ ] Pass  [ ] Fail

Student's Signature_____ Date_____

Instructor's Signature_____ Date_____

© 1992 J.B. Lippincott Company, Fundamentals of Nursing: Human Health and Function

## PROCEDURE 30-4
# SUCTIONING OROPHARYNGEAL AND NASOPHARYNGEAL AREAS

|  | E | S | U |
|---|---|---|---|
| 1. Wash hands. | [ ] | [ ] | [ ] |
| 2. Explain procedure and purpose to patient. | [ ] | [ ] | [ ] |
| 3a. Position the patient with an intact gag reflex in semi-Fowler's position. | [ ] | [ ] | [ ] |
| OR |  |  |  |
| 3b. Position the unconscious patient in side-lying position. | [ ] | [ ] | [ ] |
| 4. Turn suction device on and adjust pressure; infants and children, 50 to 75 mm Hg; adults 100 to 120 mm Hg. | [ ] | [ ] | [ ] |
| 5. Open and prepare sterile suction catheter kit: |  |  |  |
| a. Unfold sterile cup, touching only the outside. Place on bedside table. | [ ] | [ ] | [ ] |
| b. Pour approximately 100 mL sterile NaCl into cup. | [ ] | [ ] | [ ] |
| c. Put on sterile gloves. | [ ] | [ ] | [ ] |
| d. If kit supplies one glove only, place on dominant hand after donning clean glove on nondominant hand. | [ ] | [ ] | [ ] |
| 6. Pick up catheter with dominant hand. Pick up connecting tubing with nondominant hand. Attach catheter to tubing without contaminating sterile hand. | [ ] | [ ] | [ ] |
| 7. Place catheter end into cup of NaCl. Test functioning of equipment by applying thumb from nondominant hand over open port to create suction. | [ ] | [ ] | [ ] |
| 8. If patient is using an oxygen delivery system, remove with nondominant hand. | [ ] | [ ] | [ ] |
| 9. Without applying suction, insert catheter gently into nostril, directing slightly downward. If one nostril is not patent, do not force, try other nare. Advance catheter into pharynx. | [ ] | [ ] | [ ] |
| 10. Apply suction by placing thumb of non-dominant hand over open port. Rotate catheter with your dominant hand as you withdraw the catheter. This should take 5 to 10 seconds. | [ ] | [ ] | [ ] |
| 11. If patient is using supplemental oxygen, replace for several minutes between subsequent suction passes. If not using supplemental oxygen, allow 1 to 2 minutes for ventilation between subsequent passes. Encourage deep breathing. | [ ] | [ ] | [ ] |
| 12. Rinse catheter thoroughly with NaCl. | [ ] | [ ] | [ ] |
| 13. Repeat steps 9 to 12 until nasopharynx is clear. | [ ] | [ ] | [ ] |
| 14. Without applying suction, insert the catheter gently along one side of the mouth. Advance to the oropharynx. | [ ] | [ ] | [ ] |

*(continued)*

© 1992 J.B. Lippincott Company, Fundamentals of Nursing: Human Health and Function

### 30-4: Suctioning Oropharyngeal And Nasopharyngeal Areas *(Continued)*

|  | E | S | U |
|---|---|---|---|
| 15. Apply suction for 5 to 10 seconds as you rotate and withdraw the catheter. | [ ] | [ ] | [ ] |
| 16. Allow 1 to 2 minutes between passes for the patient to ventilate. Encourage deep breathing. Replace oxygen if applicable. | [ ] | [ ] | [ ] |
| 17. Repeat steps 14 and 15 as necessary to clear oropharynx. | [ ] | [ ] | [ ] |
| 18. Rinse catheter and tubing by suctioning NaCl through the catheter. | [ ] | [ ] | [ ] |
| 19. Remove gloves by holding catheter with dominant hand and pulling glove off inside out. Catheter will remain coiled inside glove. Pull other glove off inside out. Dispose of in trash receptacle. | [ ] | [ ] | [ ] |
| 20. Turn off suction device. | [ ] | [ ] | [ ] |
| 21. Assist patient to comfortable position. Offer assistance with oral and nasal hygiene. Replace oxygen delivery system if used. | [ ] | [ ] | [ ] |
| 22. Dispose of disposable supplies. | [ ] | [ ] | [ ] |
| 23. Wash hands. | [ ] | [ ] | [ ] |
| 24. Ensure that sterile suction kit is available at head of bed. | [ ] | [ ] | [ ] |
| 25. Document procedure and observations. | [ ] | [ ] | [ ] |

E = Excels;  S = Satisfactory;  U = Unsatisfactory

COMMENTS:

[ ] Pass  [ ] Fail

Student's Signature_____ Date_____

Instructor's Signature_____ Date _____

© 1992 J.B. Lippincott Company, Fundamentals of Nursing: Human Health and Function

# PROCEDURE 30-5
## SUCTIONING NASOTRACHEAL SECRETIONS

|  |  | E | S | U |
|---|---|---|---|---|
| 1. | Gather equipment. | [ ] | [ ] | [ ] |
| 2. | Wash hands. | [ ] | [ ] | [ ] |
| 3. | Explain procedure and purpose to patient. | [ ] | [ ] | [ ] |
| 4a. | Position the conscious patient with intact gag reflex in semi- or high-Fowler's position. | [ ] | [ ] | [ ] |
|  | OR |  |  |  |
| 4b. | Position the unconscious patient in side-lying position facing you. | [ ] | [ ] | [ ] |
| 5. | Turn suction device on and adjust pressure; infants and children, 50 to 75 mm Hg.; adults, 100 to 120 mm Hg. | [ ] | [ ] | [ ] |
| 6. | In accordance with agency policy and physician's orders, place oxygen mask or resuscitator bag over patient's nose and mouth. Have patient take several deep breaths. | [ ] | [ ] | [ ] |
| 7. | Open and prepare sterile suction catheter kit while patient deep-breathes. | [ ] | [ ] | [ ] |
|  | a. Unfold sterile cup, touching only the outside. Place on bedside table. | [ ] | [ ] | [ ] |
|  | b. Pour approximately 100 mL sterile NaCl into cup. | [ ] | [ ] | [ ] |
|  | c. Put on sterile gloves. If kit provides only one glove, place on dominant hand after donning clean glove on nondominant hand. | [ ] | [ ] | [ ] |
| 8. | Pick up catheter with dominant hand and attach to suction tubing without contaminating sterile hand. | [ ] | [ ] | [ ] |
| 9. | Place catheter end into NaCl. Test functioning of equipment by applying thumb from nondominant hand over open port to create suction. | [ ] | [ ] | [ ] |
| 10. | Remove oxygen delivery device with non-dominant hand. | [ ] | [ ] | [ ] |
| 11. | Without applying suction, gently insert catheter into nares using slight downward slant, or alongside and through mouth. | [ ] | [ ] | [ ] |
| 12. | Advance catheter into trachea during inspiratory phase of respiratory cycle. In adults, insert catheter 20 to 24 cm; adolescents, 14 to 20 cm; children and infants, 8 to 14 cm. | [ ] | [ ] | [ ] |
| 13. | If resistance is felt when catheter is inserted the recommended distance, pull back 1 cm before applying suction. | [ ] | [ ] | [ ] |
| 14. | Apply suction by placing thumb of non-dominant hand over open port. Rotate catheter with your dominant hand as you withdraw the catheter. This should take 5 to 10 seconds. | [ ] | [ ] | [ ] |
| 15. | Replace supplemental oxygen. Encourage deep breathing and coughing. Allow several minutes of ventilation between suction passes. | [ ] | [ ] | [ ] |

*(continued)*

© 1992 J.B. Lippincott Company, Fundamentals of Nursing: Human Health and Function

### 30-5: Suctioning Nasotracheal Secretions *(Continued)*

|  | E | S | U |
|---|---|---|---|
| 16. Monitor for alterations in cardiopulmonary status (bronchospasm, hypoxia, cardiac arrhythmias). | [ ] | [ ] | [ ] |
| 17. Rinse catheter with NaCl (saline) until clear. | [ ] | [ ] | [ ] |
| 18. Repeat steps 11 to 17 until trachea is clear of secretions. | [ ] | [ ] | [ ] |
| 19. Perform nasopharyngeal or oropharyngeal suctioning to clear secretions from upper airway. | [ ] | [ ] | [ ] |
| 20. Remove gloves by holding catheter with dominant hand and pulling glove off inside out. Catheter will remain coiled inside the glove. Pull other glove off inside out. Dispose of in trash receptacle. | [ ] | [ ] | [ ] |
| 21. Turn off suction device. | [ ] | [ ] | [ ] |
| 22. Assist patient to comfortable position. Offer assistance with nasal and oral hygiene. | [ ] | [ ] | [ ] |
| 23. Dispose of disposable supplies. | [ ] | [ ] | [ ] |
| 24. Wash hands. | [ ] | [ ] | [ ] |
| 25. Ensure that new sterile suction kit is available at head of bed. | [ ] | [ ] | [ ] |
| 26. Document procedure and observations. | [ ] | [ ] | [ ] |

E = Excels;  S = Satisfactory;  U = Unsatisfactory

COMMENTS:

[ ] Pass  [ ] Fail

Student's Signature_____ Date_____

Instructor's Signature_____ Date _____

© 1992 J.B. Lippincott Company, Fundamentals of Nursing: Human Health and Function

## PROCEDURE 30-6
## PROVIDING TRACHEOSTOMY CARE

|  | E | S | U |
|---|---|---|---|
| 1. Gather equipment. | [ ] | [ ] | [ ] |
| 2. Wash hands. | [ ] | [ ] | [ ] |
| 3. Explain procedure and purpose to patient. Place in semi- to high-Fowler's position. | [ ] | [ ] | [ ] |
| 4. Suction tracheostomy tube. Before discarding gloves, remove soiled tracheostomy dressing, and discard with catheter inside glove. | [ ] | [ ] | [ ] |
|    a. Turn suction device on and adjust pressure; infants and children, 50 to 75 mm Hg; adults, 100 to 120 mm Hg. | [ ] | [ ] | [ ] |
|    b. Open and prepare sterile suction catheter kit (as in Procedure 30-5). | [ ] | [ ] | [ ] |
|    c. Pick up catheter with dominant hand and attach to suction tubing without contaminating sterile hand. | [ ] | [ ] | [ ] |
|    d. Place catheter end into NaCl. Test functioning of equipment by applying thumb from nondominant hand over open port to create suction. | [ ] | [ ] | [ ] |
|    e. Without applying suction, gently insert catheter through tracheostomy tube and advance about 10 to 12 cm in adult. | [ ] | [ ] | [ ] |
|    f. Apply suction by placing thumb of non-dominant hand over open port. Rotate catheter with your dominant hand as you withdraw the catheter. This should take 5 to 10 seconds. | [ ] | [ ] | [ ] |
| 5. Replace oxygen or humidification source and encourage patient to deep-breathe as you prepare sterile supplies. | [ ] | [ ] | [ ] |
| 6. Open sterile tracheostomy kit. Pour normal saline into one basin, hydrogen peroxide into the second. Open several sterile cotton-tipped applicators and one sterile precut tracheostomy dressing and place on sterile field. If kit does not contain twill tape, cut two 15 inch ties and set aside. | [ ] | [ ] | [ ] |
| 7. Don sterile gloves. Maintain sterility of dominant hand throughout procedure. | [ ] | [ ] | [ ] |
| 8. Remove oxygen or humidity source. For tracheostomy tube with inner cannula, complete steps 9 to 26. For tracheostomy tube without inner cannula or plugged with a button, complete steps 14 to 26. | [ ] | [ ] | [ ] |
| 9. Unlock inner cannula by turning counter-clockwise. Remove inner cannula and place in basin with hydrogen peroxide. | [ ] | [ ] | [ ] |
| 10. Replace oxygen source over or near outer cannula, if needed. | [ ] | [ ] | [ ] |
| 11. Clean lumen and sides of inner cannula using pipe cleaners or sterile brush. | [ ] | [ ] | [ ] |

*(continued)*

© 1992 J.B. Lippincott Company, Fundamentals of Nursing: Human Health and Function

**30-6:  Providing Tracheostomy Care** *(Continued)*

| | E | S | U |
|---|---|---|---|
| 12. Rinse inner cannula thoroughly by agitating in normal saline for several seconds. | [ ] | [ ] | [ ] |
| 13. Remove oxygen source and replace inner cannula into outer cannula.  "Lock" by turning clockwise until the two blue dots align.  Replace oxygen or humidity source. | [ ] | [ ] | [ ] |
| 14. Clean stoma under faceplate with circular motion using hydrogen peroxide-soaked cotton-tipped applicators.  Cleanse dried secretions from all exposed outer cannula surfaces. | [ ] | [ ] | [ ] |
| 15. Remove foaming secretions using normal saline-soaked cotton-tipped applicators. | [ ] | [ ] | [ ] |
| 16. Pat moist surfaces dry with 4" x 4" gauze. | [ ] | [ ] | [ ] |
| 17. Place dry, sterile, precut tracheostomy dressing around tracheostomy stoma and under faceplate.  Does not use cut 4" x 4" gauze. | [ ] | [ ] | [ ] |
| 18. If tracheostomy ties are to be changed, have an assistant don a sterile glove to hold the tracheostomy tube in place. | [ ] | [ ] | [ ] |
| 19. Cut a 1/2" slit approximately 1" from one end of both clean tracheostomy ties. | [ ] | [ ] | [ ] |
| 20. Remove and discard soiled tracheostomy ties. | [ ] | [ ] | [ ] |
| 21. Thread the slit end of one clean tie through the one eyelet of the faceplate.  Thread the other end of the tie through the slit and pull it taut against the faceplate. | [ ] | [ ] | [ ] |
| 22. Repeat step 21 with the second tie. | [ ] | [ ] | [ ] |
| 23. Bring both ties together at one side of patient's neck.  Assess that ties are only tight enough to allow one finger between tie and neck.  Use two square knots to secure the ties. Trim excess tie length. | [ ] | [ ] | [ ] |
| 24. Remove gloves and discard disposable equipment.  Label, date, and store reusable supplies. | [ ] | [ ] | [ ] |
| 25. Assist patient to comfortable position and offer oral hygiene. | [ ] | [ ] | [ ] |
| 26. Wash hands. | [ ] | [ ] | [ ] |
| 27. Document procedure and observations. | [ ] | [ ] | [ ] |

E = Excels;  S = Satisfactory;  U = Unsatisfactory

COMMENTS:

[ ] Pass  [ ] Fail

Student's Signature_____  Date_____

Instructor's Signature_____  Date _____

© 1992 J.B. Lippincott Company, Fundamentals of Nursing:  Human Health and Function

### PROCEDURE 30-7A
# MANAGING AN OBSTRUCTED AIRWAY IN A CONSCIOUS ADULT
## (HEIMLICH MANEUVER)

|  |  | E | S | U |
|---|---|---|---|---|
| 1. | Assess patient. | [ ] | [ ] | [ ] |
| 2. | The patient is standing or sitting. | [ ] | [ ] | [ ] |
| 3. | Stand behind patient. | [ ] | [ ] | [ ] |
| 4. | Wrap your arms around patient's waist. | [ ] | [ ] | [ ] |
| 5. | Make a fist with one hand.  Place thumb side of fist against patient's abdomen, above navel but below the xiphoid process. | [ ] | [ ] | [ ] |
| 6. | Grasp fist with other hand. | [ ] | [ ] | [ ] |
| 7. | Press fist into abdomen with a quick upward thrust. | [ ] | [ ] | [ ] |
| 8. | Repeat distinct separate thrusts until foreign body is expelled or patient becomes unconscious. | [ ] | [ ] | [ ] |

E = Excels;  S = Satisfactory;  U = Unsatisfactory

COMMENTS:

[ ] Pass  [ ] Fail

Student's Signature_____ Date_____

Instructor's Signature_____ Date _____

© 1992 J.B. Lippincott Company, Fundamentals of Nursing:  Human Health and Function

# PROCEDURE 30-7B
# MANAGING AN OBSTRUCTED AIRWAY IN
# AN UNCONSCIOUS ADULT
# (HEIMLICH MANEUVER)
## (Abdominal Thrust)

|  | E | S | U |
|---|---|---|---|
| 1. Assess patient. Patient will be lying on the ground. | [ ] | [ ] | [ ] |
| 2. Turn patient on back and call for help. | [ ] | [ ] | [ ] |
| 3. Finger sweep (avoid in infants and children):<br>a. Use tongue-jaw lift to open mouth. | [ ] | [ ] | [ ] |
| b. Insert index finger inside cheek and sweep to base of tongue. Use a hooking motion if possible to dislodge and remove foreign body. | [ ] | [ ] | [ ] |
| 4. Straddle patient's thighs or kneel to the side of thighs. | [ ] | [ ] | [ ] |
| 5. Place heel of one hand on epigastric area, midline above the navel but below the xiphoid process. | [ ] | [ ] | [ ] |
| 6. Place second hand on top of first hand. | [ ] | [ ] | [ ] |
| 7. Press heel of hand into abdomen with quick upward thrust in the midline. | [ ] | [ ] | [ ] |
| 8. Repeat abdominal thrusts 6 to 10 times. | [ ] | [ ] | [ ] |
| 9. If airway is still obstructed, attempt to ventilate using mouth-to-mouth respiration and head tilt-chin lift. | [ ] | [ ] | [ ] |
| 10. Repeat steps 5 to 8 until successful. | [ ] | [ ] | [ ] |

E = Excels;  S = Satisfactory;  U = Unsatisfactory

COMMENTS:

[ ] Pass  [ ] Fail

Student's Signature_____ Date_____

Instructor's Signature_____ Date_____

© 1992 J.B. Lippincott Company, Fundamentals of Nursing: Human Health and Function

88

## PROCEDURE 30-7C
## MANAGING AN OBSTRUCTED AIRWAY IN INFANTS
## UNDER 1 YEAR OF AGE
### (Back Blows and Chest Thrusts)

|  |  | E | S | U |
|---|---|---|---|---|
| 1. | Assess patient. | [ ] | [ ] | [ ] |
| 2. | Straddle infant over your arm with head lower than trunk. | [ ] | [ ] | [ ] |
| 3. | Support head by holding jaw firmly in your hand. | [ ] | [ ] | [ ] |
| 4. | Rest your forearm on your thigh and deliver four back blows with the heel of your hand between the infant's scapula. | [ ] | [ ] | [ ] |
| 5. | Place free hand on infant's back and support neck while turning to supine position. | [ ] | [ ] | [ ] |
| 6. | Place two fingers over sternum in same location as for external chest compression (one fingerwidth below nipple line). | [ ] | [ ] | [ ] |
| 7. | Administer four chest thrusts. | [ ] | [ ] | [ ] |
| 8. | Repeat steps 2 to 7 until airway is not obstructed. | [ ] | [ ] | [ ] |

E = Excels;  S = Satisfactory;  U = Unsatisfactory

COMMENTS:

[ ] Pass  [ ] Fail

Student's Signature_____ Date_____

Instructor's Signature_____ Date _____

© 1992 J.B. Lippincott Company, Fundamentals of Nursing: Human Health and Function

# PROCEDURE 30-7D
# MANAGING AN OBSTRUCTED AIRWAY IN CHILDREN
# OVER 1 YEAR OF AGE

|  |  | E | S | U |
|---|---|---|---|---|
| 1. | Assess patient. | [ ] | [ ] | [ ] |
| 2. | Perform Heimlich maneuver with child standing, sitting, or lying as for adult, but more gently. | [ ] | [ ] | [ ] |
| 3. | Rescuer kneels behind child or has child stand on table. | [ ] | [ ] | [ ] |
| 4. | Prevent foreign body airway obstruction in infants and children by teaching parents and caregivers to: |  |  |  |
|  | a. Restrict children from walking, running, or playing with food or foreign objects in their mouths. | [ ] | [ ] | [ ] |
|  | b. Keep small objects (i.e. marbles, beads, beans, thumb tacks) away from children under 3 years of age. | [ ] | [ ] | [ ] |
|  | c. Avoid feeding popcorn and peanuts to children under 3 years of age, and cut other foods into small pieces. | [ ] | [ ] | [ ] |
| 5. | Teach parents and caregivers the management of foreign body airway obstruction. | [ ] | [ ] | [ ] |

E = Excels;  S = Satisfactory;  U = Unsatisfactory

COMMENTS:

[ ] Pass  [ ] Fail

Student's Signature_____ Date_____

Instructor's Signature_____ Date _____

© 1992 J.B. Lippincott Company, Fundamentals of Nursing: Human Health and Function

## PROCEDURE 30-7E
# MANAGING AN OBSTRUCTED AIRWAY IN PREGNANT WOMEN
# OR VERY OBESE ADULTS
### (Chest Thrusts)

|  |  | E | S | U |
|---|---|---|---|---|
| 1. | Assess patient. | [ ] | [ ] | [ ] |
| 2. | Stand behind patient. | [ ] | [ ] | [ ] |
| 3. | Bring your arms under patient's armpits and around chest. | [ ] | [ ] | [ ] |
| 4. | Make a fist and place thumb side against middle of sternum. | [ ] | [ ] | [ ] |
| 5. | Grasp fist with other hand and deliver a quick backward thrust. | [ ] | [ ] | [ ] |
| 6. | Repeat thrusts until airway is cleared. | [ ] | [ ] | [ ] |
| 7. | If patient is supine, perform chest thrusts with hands positioned with heel over lower half of sternum (as for cardiac compression). Administer separate downward thrusts until airway is cleared. | [ ] | [ ] | [ ] |

E = Excels;  S = Satisfactory;  U = Unsatisfactory

COMMENTS:

[ ] Pass  [ ] Fail

Student's Signature_____ Date_____

Instructor's Signature_____ Date _____

© 1992 J.B. Lippincott Company, Fundamentals of Nursing: Human Health and Function

## PROCEDURE 31-1
## APPLYING ANTIEMBOLIC STOCKINGS

|  | E | S | U |
|---|---|---|---|
| 1. Gather equipment. | [ ] | [ ] | [ ] |
| 2. Wash hands. | [ ] | [ ] | [ ] |
| 3. Explain procedure and purpose to patient. | [ ] | [ ] | [ ] |
| 4. Position patient in supine position for one half hour before applying stockings. | [ ] | [ ] | [ ] |
| 5. Provide privacy for patient. | [ ] | [ ] | [ ] |
| 6. Gather material from length of stocking down to the toe. | [ ] | [ ] | [ ] |
| 7. Ease the stocking over the patient's toe and heel and adjust to fit snugly. | [ ] | [ ] | [ ] |
| 8. Gently pull the stocking over the leg removing all wrinkles. | [ ] | [ ] | [ ] |
| 9. Assess toes for circulation and warmth. Check area at top of stocking for binding. | [ ] | [ ] | [ ] |
| 10. Remove antiembolic stockings at least twice daily. | [ ] | [ ] | [ ] |

E = Excels;  S = Satisfactory;  U = Unsatisfactory

COMMENTS:

[ ] Pass  [ ] Fail

Student's Signature_____ Date_____

Instructor's Signature_____ Date_____

© 1992 J.B. Lippincott Company, Fundamentals of Nursing: Human Health and Function

## PROCEDURE 31-2A
# ADMINISTERING CARDIOPULMONARY RESUSCITATION (CPR)
## ONE RESCUER - ADULT PATIENT

|  | | E | S | U |
|---|---|---|---|---|
| 1. | Assess to determine responsiveness. Shake gently. | [ ] | [ ] | [ ] |
| 2. | Call for help. | [ ] | [ ] | [ ] |
| 3. | Turn patient onto back while supporting head and neck. Place a cardiac board under back or place patient on floor. | [ ] | [ ] | [ ] |
| 4. | Open the airway using a head tilt/chin lift. | [ ] | [ ] | [ ] |
| 5. | Place your ear over patient's mouth, and observe the chest for rising with respiration. Listen, look, and feel for breathing for 3 to 5 seconds. | [ ] | [ ] | [ ] |
| 6. | Pinch the patient's nostrils with thumb and index finger of hand holding the forehead. | [ ] | [ ] | [ ] |
| 7. | Take a deep breath and place your mouth around the patient's mouth with a tight seal. | [ ] | [ ] | [ ] |
| 8. | Ventilate two full breaths. Each breath takes 1 to 1.5 seconds to deliver. Pause between breaths to allow for lung deflation and to take another deep breath. | [ ] | [ ] | [ ] |
| 9. | Assess for carotid pulse for 5 seconds on the side next to which you are kneeling. Maintain head tilt with other hand. | [ ] | [ ] | [ ] |
| 10. | If patient is pulseless: call for help. | [ ] | [ ] | [ ] |
| 11. | With hand nearest patient's legs, place middle and index fingers on lower ridge of near ribs and move fingers up along ribs to costal-sternal notch in center of lower chest. | [ ] | [ ] | [ ] |
| 12. | Place middle finger on this notch and index finger next to the middle finger on the lower end of the notch. | [ ] | [ ] | [ ] |
| 13. | Place heel of other hand along the lower half of the sternum, next to the index finger. | [ ] | [ ] | [ ] |
| 14. | Remove first hand from the notch and place heel of that hand parallel over the hand on the chest. Interlock fingers, keeping them off patient's chest. | [ ] | [ ] | [ ] |
| 15. | Keeping your hands on sternum, extend your arms, locking the elbows, with your shoulders directly over the patient's chest. | [ ] | [ ] | [ ] |
| 16. | Press down on chest, depressing sternum 1.5 to 2 inches. | [ ] | [ ] | [ ] |
| 17. | Completely release compression while maintaining your hand position. Repeat in a smooth rhythm 80 to 100 times/minute. | [ ] | [ ] | [ ] |
| 18. | Ventilate with 2 full breaths after every 15 chest compressions. | [ ] | [ ] | [ ] |

*(continued)*

© 1992 J.B. Lippincott Company, Fundamentals of Nursing: Human Health and Function

**31-2:  Administering Cardiopulmonary Resuscitation (CPR)**
**One Rescuer - Adult Patient** *(Continued)*

|  | E | S | U |
|---|---|---|---|
| 19. Repeat 4 cycles of 15 chest compressions and 2 ventilations. | [ ] | [ ] | [ ] |
| 20. Reassess for carotid pulse.  If patient is pulseless, continue CPR.  Reassess for carotid pulse every few minutes without interrupting CPR for longer than 7 seconds. | [ ] | [ ] | [ ] |

E = Excels;  S = Satisfactory;  U = Unsatisfactory

COMMENTS:

[ ] Pass  [ ] Fail

Student's Signature_____  Date_____

Instructor's Signature_____  Date _____

© 1992 J.B. Lippincott Company, Fundamentals of Nursing:  Human Health and Function

# PROCEDURE 31-2B
# ADMINISTERING CARDIOPULMONARY RESUSCITATION (CPR)
## TWO RESCUERS - ADULT PATIENT

|  | E | S | U |
|---|---|---|---|
| 1. Assess to determine responsiveness.  Shake gently. | [ ] | [ ] | [ ] |
| 2. Call for help. | [ ] | [ ] | [ ] |
| 3. Turn patient onto back while supporting head and neck.  Place a cardiac board under back or place patient on floor. | [ ] | [ ] | [ ] |
| 4. Open the airway using a head tilt/chin lift. | [ ] | [ ] | [ ] |
| 5. Place your ear over patient's mouth, and observe the chest for rising with respiration. <u>Listen, look, and feel</u> for breathing for 3 to 5 seconds. | [ ] | [ ] | [ ] |
| 6. Pinch the patient's nostrils with thumb and index finger of hand holding the forehead. | [ ] | [ ] | [ ] |
| 7. Take a deep breath and place your mouth around the patient's mouth with a tight seal. | [ ] | [ ] | [ ] |
| 8. Ventilate two full breaths.  Each breath takes 1 to 1.5 seconds to deliver.  Pause between breaths to allow for lung deflation and to take another deep breath. | [ ] | [ ] | [ ] |
| 9. Assess for carotid pulse for 5 seconds on the side next to which you are kneeling.  Maintain head tilt with other hand. | [ ] | [ ] | [ ] |
| 10. If patient is pulseless:  call for help. | [ ] | [ ] | [ ] |
| 11. With hand nearest patient's legs, place middle and index fingers on lower ridge of near ribs and move fingers up along ribs to costal-sternal notch in center of lower chest. | [ ] | [ ] | [ ] |
| 12. Place middle finger on this notch and index finger next to the middle finger on the lower end of the notch. | [ ] | [ ] | [ ] |
| 13. Place heel of other hand along the lower half of the sternum, next to the index finger. | [ ] | [ ] | [ ] |
| 14. Remove first hand from the notch and place heel of that hand parallel over the hand on the chest.  Interlock fingers, keeping them off patient's chest. | [ ] | [ ] | [ ] |
| 15. Keeping your hands on sternum, extend your arms, locking the elbows, with your shoulders directly over the patient's chest. | [ ] | [ ] | [ ] |
| 16. Press down on chest, depressing sternum 1.5 to 2 inches. | [ ] | [ ] | [ ] |
| 17. Completely release compression while maintaining your hand position.  Repeat in a smooth rhythm 80 to 100 times/minute. | [ ] | [ ] | [ ] |
| 18. Ventilate with 2 full breaths after every 15 chest compressions. | [ ] | [ ] | [ ] |
| 19. Repeat 4 cycles of 15 chest compressions and 2 ventilations. | [ ] | [ ] | [ ] |
| 20. Reassess for carotid pulse.  If patient is pulseless, continue CPR.  Reassess for carotid pulse every few minutes without interrupting CPR for longer than 7 seconds. | [ ] | [ ] | [ ] |

*(continued)*

© 1992 J.B. Lippincott Company, Fundamentals of Nursing:  Human Health and Function

31-2B:   **Administering Cardiopulmonary Resuscitation (CPR)**
         **Two Rescuers - Adult Patient**  *(Continued)*

|  |  | E | S | U |
|---|---|---|---|---|
| 21. | When second rescuer arrives, the first rescuer stops CPR after completing two ventilations and assesses for carotid pulse for 5 seconds. | [ ] | [ ] | [ ] |
| 22. | The second rescuer moves into the chest compression position. | [ ] | [ ] | [ ] |
| 23. | If pulselessness continues, the first rescuer states "no pulse" and delivers one ventilation. | [ ] | [ ] | [ ] |
| 24. | Second rescuer begins chest compression while counting out loud, "one and two and three and four and five and ..." The compression rate is 80 to 100/minute. | [ ] | [ ] | [ ] |
| 25. | First rescuer gives one full ventilation after every 5 chest compressions.  First rescuer also assesses carotid pulse during chest compressions to evaluate effectiveness. | [ ] | [ ] | [ ] |
| 26. | When second rescuer wishes to change positions, he or she states "Change, one and two and three and four and five and". | [ ] | [ ] | [ ] |
| 27. | First rescuer delivers the ventilation then moves into the chest compression position. | [ ] | [ ] | [ ] |
| 28. | Second rescuer moves to the ventilator position and assesses for carotid pulse for 5 seconds.  If pulseless, resume CPR. | [ ] | [ ] | [ ] |

E = Excels;  S = Satisfactory;  U = Unsatisfactory

**COMMENTS:**

[ ] Pass  [ ] Fail

Student's Signature_____   Date_____

Instructor's Signature_____   Date _____

© 1992 J.B. Lippincott Company, Fundamentals of Nursing:  Human Health and Function

96

## PROCEDURE 31-2C
# ADMINISTERING CARDIOPULMONARY RESUSCITATION (CPR)
## ONE RESCUER - INFANT AND CHILD PATIENT

|  | E | S | U |
|---|---|---|---|
| 1. Assess for unresponsiveness. Shake gently. | [ ] | [ ] | [ ] |
| 2. Call for help. | [ ] | [ ] | [ ] |
| 3. Place child on hard surface. | [ ] | [ ] | [ ] |
| 4. Open the airway using head tilt/chin lift. Avoid overextension of head in infants. | [ ] | [ ] | [ ] |
| 5. Place your ear over child's mouth and observe chest for rise. Listen, look, and feel for breathing. | [ ] | [ ] | [ ] |
| 6. Perform Heimlich maneuver if airway obstruction from food or foreign object is suspected. | [ ] | [ ] | [ ] |
| 7. If breathlessness is determined, seal mouth and nose and ventilate twice (1 to 1.5 seconds for each breath). Observe for chest rise. | [ ] | [ ] | [ ] |
| 8. Assess pulselessness by palpating for carotid artery on near side of children over 1 year of age. In infants less than 1 year, assess brachial pulse for 5 seconds. | [ ] | [ ] | [ ] |
| 9. Begin chest compression if pulseless. For infant up to 1 year: |  |  |  |
|    a. Visualize an imaginary line between the infant's nipples. | [ ] | [ ] | [ ] |
|    b. Place index finger on sternum just below imaginary line. | [ ] | [ ] | [ ] |
|    c. Place middle and fourth fingers on sternum next to index finger. | [ ] | [ ] | [ ] |

**OR**

|  | E | S | U |
|---|---|---|---|
| 10. Begin chest compression if pulseless. For child 1 to 8 years of age: |  |  |  |
|    a. Place hand on sternum same as for adult CPR. Use one hand to compress sternum 1.5 inches 80 to 100 times/minute. | [ ] | [ ] | [ ] |
|    b. Continue chest compressions and ventilate at the rate of one breath to five compressions. | [ ] | [ ] | [ ] |
|    c. Continue CPR as for an adult. | [ ] | [ ] | [ ] |

E = Excels; S = Satisfactory; U = Unsatisfactory

COMMENTS:

[ ] Pass  [ ] Fail

Student's Signature_____ Date_____

Instructor's Signature_____ Date _____

# PROCEDURE 32-1
## MONITORING AN INTRAVENOUS INFUSION

|  |  | E | S | U |
|---|---|:---:|:---:|:---:|
| 1. | Gather equipment. | [ ] | [ ] | [ ] |
| 2. | Compare intravenous fluid currently infusing with the ordered solution. | [ ] | [ ] | [ ] |
| 3. | Inspect the rate of flow at least every hour. Check actual flow rate for 15 seconds and compare with prescribed rate of flow. If infusion is ahead of schedule, slow it so the infusion will complete at the planned time. If infusion is behind schedule, review hospital policy before increasing flow rate. | [ ] | [ ] | [ ] |
| 4. | Inspect the system for leakage and, if present, locate the source. Tighten all connections within the system. If leak is still present, slow IV flow rate to keep vein open and replace tubing with sterile set. | [ ] | [ ] | [ ] |
| 5. | Inspect the tubing for kinks or blockages. Tubing should be loosely coiled and placed on bed. | [ ] | [ ] | [ ] |
| 6. | Observe the fluid level in drip chamber. If it is less than half full, squeeze the chamber gently to allow more fluid in. | [ ] | [ ] | [ ] |
| 7. | Inspect the infusion site for signs of infiltration: decreased rate of flow, swelling, pallor, coolness, and discomfort at or above needle site. If present, the IV site is changed. If large amount of fluid infiltrated, elevate arm above heart on several pillows. | [ ] | [ ] | [ ] |
| 8. | Inspect arm above the insertion site for signs of phlebitis, inflammation of the vein: redness, swelling, warmth and pain along the vein above the IV insertion site. If present, IV is discontinued and restarted in another area. | [ ] | [ ] | [ ] |
| 9. | Inspect the insertion site for bleeding. | [ ] | [ ] | [ ] |
| 10. | If patient is able to comply, teach to contact nurse if: | [ ] | [ ] | [ ] |

- Flow rate changes suddenly.
- Fluid container is almost empty.
- Blood is in tubing.
- Site becomes uncomfortable.

| 11. | Chart any findings indicating complications of intravenous therapy (e.g. infiltration). | [ ] | [ ] | [ ] |

E = Excels; S = Satisfactory; U = Unsatisfactory

COMMENTS:


[ ] Pass  [ ] Fail

Student's Signature_____ Date_____

Instructor's Signature_____ Date _____

© 1992 J.B. Lippincott Company, Fundamentals of Nursing: Human Health and Function

## PROCEDURE 32-2A
## CHANGING INTRAVENOUS SOLUTION CONTAINER

|  |  | E | S | U |
|---|---|---|---|---|
| 1. | Gather equipment. | [ ] | [ ] | [ ] |
| 2. | Wash hands. | [ ] | [ ] | [ ] |
| 3. | Explain procedure and purpose to patient. | [ ] | [ ] | [ ] |
| 4. | Compare solution with physician's order. | [ ] | [ ] | [ ] |
| 5. | Label solution container with patient's name, solution type, additives, date, and time hung. Time label side of container. Record solution change. | [ ] | [ ] | [ ] |
| 6. | Prepare container for spiking:<br>a. If solution is in a plastic bag, remove plastic cover from entry nipple. Maintain sterility of nipple end. | [ ] | [ ] | [ ] |
|  | b. If solution is in a bottle, remove metal cap, metal disk, and rubber disk. Maintain sterility of bottle top. | [ ] | [ ] | [ ] |
| 7. | Close clamp on existing tubing. | [ ] | [ ] | [ ] |
| 8. | Take old solution container from IV pole and invert it. | [ ] | [ ] | [ ] |
| 9. | Remove spike from used container, maintaining its sterility. Spike new intravenous container with firm push/twist motion. | [ ] | [ ] | [ ] |
| 10. | Hang new container on IV pole. | [ ] | [ ] | [ ] |
| 11. | Inspect tubing for air bubbles and assess that drip chamber is one-half full of solution. | [ ] | [ ] | [ ] |
| 12. | Adjust clamp to regulate flow rate, according to the physician's order. | [ ] | [ ] | [ ] |

E = Excels; S = Satisfactory; U = Unsatisfactory

COMMENTS:

[ ] Pass [ ] Fail

Student's Signature_____ Date_____

Instructor's Signature_____ Date_____

© 1992 J.B. Lippincott Company, Fundamentals of Nursing: Human Health and Function

## PROCEDURE 32-2B
## CHANGING INTRAVENOUS SOLUTION AND TUBING

|  |  | E | S | U |
|---|---|---|---|---|
| 1. | Gather equipment. | [ ] | [ ] | [ ] |
| 2. | Wash hands. | [ ] | [ ] | [ ] |
| 3. | Explain procedure and purpose to patient. | [ ] | [ ] | [ ] |
| 4. | Compare solution with physician's order. | [ ] | [ ] | [ ] |
| 5. | Label solution container with patient's name, solution type, additives, date, and time hung.  Time label side of container. | [ ] | [ ] | [ ] |
| 6. | Open new tubing package, keeping protective covers on spike and catheter adapter. | [ ] | [ ] | [ ] |
| 7. | Adjust roller clamp on new tubing to fully closed position. | [ ] | [ ] | [ ] |
| 8. | Prepare container for spiking: | | | |
| | a. If solution is in a plastic bag, remove plastic cover from entry nipple.  Maintain sterility of nipple end. | [ ] | [ ] | [ ] |
| | b. If solution is in a bottle, remove metal cap, metal disk, and rubber disk.  Maintain sterility of bottle top. | [ ] | [ ] | [ ] |
| 9. | Remove protective cover from spike, maintaining sterility, and spike into new solution container. | [ ] | [ ] | [ ] |
| 10. | Hang container and "prime" drip chamber by squeezing gently, allowing to fill one-half full. | [ ] | [ ] | [ ] |
| 11. | Remove protective cap from catheter adapter and adjust roller clamp to flush tubing with fluid.  Replace protective cap. | [ ] | [ ] | [ ] |
| 12. | Adjust roller clamp on old tubing to close fully. | [ ] | [ ] | [ ] |
| 13. | Don clean disposable gloves. | [ ] | [ ] | [ ] |
| 14. | Hold catheter hub with fingers of one hand.  Remove old dressings if necessary.  Disconnect tubing using gentle twisting motion. | [ ] | [ ] | [ ] |
| 15. | Grasp new tubing, remove protective catheter cap, and insert tightly into needle hub, while continuing to stabilize catheter hub with other hand. | [ ] | [ ] | [ ] |
| 16. | Adjust roller clamp to start solution flowing according to physician's order. | [ ] | [ ] | [ ] |
| 17. | Remove and discard gloves. | [ ] | [ ] | [ ] |
| 18. | Secure tubing with tape. | [ ] | [ ] | [ ] |
| 19. | If dressing was removed, apply new dressing to IV site according to agency policy. | [ ] | [ ] | [ ] |
| 20. | Label new tubing with date, time, and your initials. | [ ] | [ ] | [ ] |
| 21. | Record solution and tubing change. | [ ] | [ ] | [ ] |

E = Excels;  S = Satisfactory;  U = Unsatisfactory

COMMENTS:

[ ] Pass  [ ] Fail

Student's Signature_____ Date_____

Instructor's Signature_____ Date _____

© 1992 J.B. Lippincott Company, Fundamentals of Nursing:  Human Health and Function

100

## PROCEDURE 32-3
## ADMINISTERING A BLOOD TRANSFUSION

|  | E | S | U |
|---|---|---|---|
| 1. Gather equipment. | [ ] | [ ] | [ ] |
| 2. Wash hands. | [ ] | [ ] | [ ] |
| 3. Explain procedure and purpose to patient. Have patient sign consent form if required by agency policy. | [ ] | [ ] | [ ] |
| 4. Obtain patient's vital signs, including temperature. | [ ] | [ ] | [ ] |
| 5. With another RN at patient's bedside, verify the blood product and the patient's identity by comparing the laboratory blood record with: | [ ] | [ ] | [ ] |
| a. Patient's name and identification number. | [ ] | [ ] | [ ] |
| b. Blood unit number on the blood bag label. | [ ] | [ ] | [ ] |
| c. Blood group and RH type on the blood bag label. | [ ] | [ ] | [ ] |
| d. Verify the type of blood component and the expiration date noted on the blood label. | [ ] | [ ] | [ ] |
| e. Document verification by both RN signatures on transfusion record. | [ ] | [ ] | [ ] |
| 6. Wash hands. | [ ] | [ ] | [ ] |
| 7. Open Y-type blood administration set and clamp both rollers completely. | [ ] | [ ] | [ ] |
| 8. Spike 0.9 NaCl container. Prime drip chamber and tubing with saline. | [ ] | [ ] | [ ] |
| 9. Spike blood or blood component unit with second spike. Keep roller clamp shut. | [ ] | [ ] | [ ] |
| 10. Remove primary IV tubing from catheter hub and cover end with sterile protector. | [ ] | [ ] | [ ] |
| 11. Attach blood administration tubing to catheter hub and secure with tape. | [ ] | [ ] | [ ] |
| 12. Close clamp to 0.9 NaCl container. Open clamp to blood product. Open roller clamp below drip chamber and begin transfusion. | [ ] | [ ] | [ ] |
| 13. Infuse blood slowly for first 15 minutes at 10 drops per minute. | [ ] | [ ] | [ ] |
| 14. Monitor and document vital signs every 5 minutes during first 15 minutes, assessing for chilling, back pain, headache, nausea or vomiting, tachycardia, hypotension, tachypnea, or skin rash. | [ ] | [ ] | [ ] |
| 15. If adverse reactions occur, close clamp to blood, open clamp to 0.9 NaCl, and notify physician immediately. Follow agency policy for laboratory notification and obtaining blood and urine specimens. | [ ] | [ ] | [ ] |
| 16. If no adverse reactions occur after 15 minutes, regulate clamp to increase infusion according to physician's order. Monitor vital signs hourly until transfusion is complete. | [ ] | [ ] | [ ] |

*(continued)*

© 1992 J.B. Lippincott Company, Fundamentals of Nursing: Human Health and Function

32-3: Administering A Blood Transfusion *(Continued)*

|  | E | S | U |
|---|---|---|---|
| 17. When blood transfusion is complete, clamp roller to blood and open roller to 0.9 NaCl solution. Infuse until tubing is clear. | [ ] | [ ] | [ ] |
| 18. Obtain and document post-transfusion vital signs. | [ ] | [ ] | [ ] |
| 19. If second blood component unit is to be transfused, slow 0.9 NaCl solution to keep vein open until next unit is available. Follow verification procedure and vital sign monitoring for each unit. | [ ] | [ ] | [ ] |
| 20. If transfusion orders are complete, disconnect the blood administration tubing from catheter hub. Reconnect primary intravenous solution and tubing and adjust to desired rate. | [ ] | [ ] | [ ] |
| 21. Discard blood administration equipment according to agency policy. | [ ] | [ ] | [ ] |
| 22. Wash hands. | [ ] | [ ] | [ ] |

E = Excels;  S = Satisfactory;  U = Unsatisfactory

COMMENTS:

[ ] Pass  [ ] Fail

Student's Signature_____ Date_____

Instructor's Signature_____ Date _____

© 1992 J.B. Lippincott Company, Fundamentals of Nursing: Human Health and Function

# PROCEDURE 33-1
## ASSISTING AN ADULT WITH FEEDING

|  | | E | S | U |
|---|---|---|---|---|
| 1. | Prepare patient's environment for meal: | [ ] | [ ] | [ ] |
| | a. Remove urinal, bedpan, dressings, trash. | [ ] | [ ] | [ ] |
| | b. Ventilate or aerate room for unpleasant odors. | [ ] | [ ] | [ ] |
| | c. Clean overbed table. | [ ] | [ ] | [ ] |
| 2. | Prepare patient for meal: | [ ] | [ ] | [ ] |
| | a. Help patient to urinate or defecate. | [ ] | [ ] | [ ] |
| | b. Help patient to wash face and hands. | [ ] | [ ] | [ ] |
| | c. Assist with oral hygiene. | [ ] | [ ] | [ ] |
| | d. Help patient to apply dentures, glasses, or special appliances. | [ ] | [ ] | [ ] |
| | e. Assist to upright position in bed or chair. | [ ] | [ ] | [ ] |
| 3. | Wash hands before touching meal tray. | [ ] | [ ] | [ ] |
| 4. | Check patient's tray against diet order. | [ ] | [ ] | [ ] |
| 5. | Place tray on overbed table and move in front of patient. | [ ] | [ ] | [ ] |
| 6. | Prepare tray. Open cartons, remove lids, season food, cut food into bite-size pieces. | [ ] | [ ] | [ ] |
| 7. | Place napkin or towel under patient's chin. | [ ] | [ ] | [ ] |
| 8. | If patient can feed self, leave and return in 10 to 15 minutes to determine if patient is tolerating diet. | [ ] | [ ] | [ ] |
| 9. | If patient needs help to eat, sit in chair facing patient. If patient remains in bed, nurse stands. | [ ] | [ ] | [ ] |
| 10. | Allow patient to choose the order in which he or she would like to eat. If patient is visually impaired, identify the food on the tray. | [ ] | [ ] | [ ] |
| 11. | Warn patient if food is hot or cold. | [ ] | [ ] | [ ] |
| 12. | Allow enough time between bites for adequate chewing and swallowing. | [ ] | [ ] | [ ] |
| 13. | Offer liquids as requested or between bites. Use straw or special drinking cup if available. | [ ] | [ ] | [ ] |
| 14. | Provide conversation during meal. Choose topic of interest to patient. Reorient to current events or use meal as opportunity to educate on nutrition or discharge plans. | [ ] | [ ] | [ ] |
| 15. | Help patient to wash hands and face, and perform oral hygiene after meal. | [ ] | [ ] | [ ] |
| 16. | Assist to comfortable position and allow rest period. If at risk for aspiration, leave head of bed elevated for 30 minutes after eating. | [ ] | [ ] | [ ] |
| 17. | Record fluids and amount of meal consumed, if ordered. | [ ] | [ ] | [ ] |

*(continued)*

© 1992 J.B. Lippincott Company, Fundamentals of Nursing: Human Health and Function

**33-1: Assisting An Adult With Feeding** *(Continued)*

| | E | S | U |
|---|---|---|---|
| 18. Remove and dispose of tray. | [ ] | [ ] | [ ] |
| 19. Wash hands. | [ ] | [ ] | [ ] |

**E = Excels;  S = Satisfactory;  U = Unsatisfactory**

**COMMENTS:**

[ ] Pass  [ ] Fail

**Student's Signature**_____ Date_____

**Instructor's Signature**_____ Date _____

© 1992 J.B. Lippincott Company, Fundamentals of Nursing: Human Health and Function

104

## PROCEDURE 33-2A
## ADMINISTERING NUTRITION VIA NASOGASTRIC
## OR GASTROSTOMY TUBE
### (Bolus or Intermittent Feeding)

|  | E | S | U |
|---|---|---|---|
| 1. Gather equipment. | [ ] | [ ] | [ ] |
| 2. Wash hands. | [ ] | [ ] | [ ] |
| 3. Explain procedure and purpose to patient. | [ ] | [ ] | [ ] |
| 4. Close room door or curtains around bed. | [ ] | [ ] | [ ] |
| 5. Help patient to high-Fowler's position by elevating head of bed at least 60 degrees or assisting to chair. If high-Fowler's position is contraindicated, help patient to a right side-lying position with head slightly elevated. | [ ] | [ ] | [ ] |
| 6. Confirm placement of tube in stomach: | | | |
| a. Attach 60 mL irrigation syringe to tube and inject 10 mL of air while auscultating over epigastrium. Recognize that this may not be reliable index of tube placement if patient has small-bore feeding tube. | [ ] | [ ] | [ ] |
| b. Aspirate all stomach contents and measure residual. | [ ] | [ ] | [ ] |
| c. If 100 mL or more than half of last feeding is aspirated, contact physician before proceeding with tube feeding. | [ ] | [ ] | [ ] |
| d. Reinstill the aspirated gastric contents through tube into stomach. | [ ] | [ ] | [ ] |
| 7. Prepare correct amount and strength of formula at room temperature. | [ ] | [ ] | [ ] |
| 8. Remove plunger from irrigation syringe. Clamp gastric tubing and attach syringe. If using gavage bag, attach tubing to gastric tube. | [ ] | [ ] | [ ] |
| 9. Fill syringe or gavage bag with formula. | [ ] | [ ] | [ ] |
| 10. Allow feeding to flow in slowly over 10 to 15 minutes. If using syringe, raise and lower to adjust flow rate by gravity. Refill syringe as needed without disconnecting, avoiding air spaces in tubing. If gavage bag is used, hang bag on IV pole and adjust flow rate with clamp on tubing. | [ ] | [ ] | [ ] |
| 11. Clamp tubing just as feeding is completing. Rinse tube with 30 to 60 mL tap water. Do not allow air to enter tubing. | [ ] | [ ] | [ ] |
| 12. Clamp gastric tube and disconnect from syringe or gavage bag. | [ ] | [ ] | [ ] |
| 13. Have patient remain in high-Fowler's or elevated side-lying position for 30 to 60 minutes. | [ ] | [ ] | [ ] |
| 14. Wash any reusable equipment with soap and water. Change equipment every 24 hours or according to agency policy. | [ ] | [ ] | [ ] |

*(continued)*

© 1992 J.B. Lippincott Company, Fundamentals of Nursing: Human Health and Function

**33-2A:** **Administering Nutrition Via Nasogastric Or Gastrostomy Tube**
**(Bolus or Intermittent Feeding)** *(Continued)*

|  | E | S | U |
|---|---|---|---|
| 15. Wash hands. | [ ] | [ ] | [ ] |
| 16. Document procedure and observations. | [ ] | [ ] | [ ] |

E = Excels;  S = Satisfactory;  U = Unsatisfactory

COMMENTS:

[ ] Pass  [ ] Fail

Student's Signature_____ Date_____

Instructor's Signature_____ Date _____

© 1992 J.B. Lippincott Company, Fundamentals of Nursing:  Human Health and Function

## PROCEDURE 33-2B
# ADMINISTERING NUTRITION VIA NASOGASTRIC
# OR GASTROSTOMY TUBE
### (Continuous Feeding)

|  | | E | S | U |
|---|---|---|---|---|
| 1. | Gather equipment. | [ ] | [ ] | [ ] |
| 2. | Wash hands. | [ ] | [ ] | [ ] |
| 3. | Explain procedure and purpose to patient. | [ ] | [ ] | [ ] |
| 4. | Close room door or curtains around bed. | [ ] | [ ] | [ ] |
| 5. | Help patient to high-Fowler's position by elevating head of bed at least 60 degrees or assisting to chair. If high-Fowler's position is contraindicated, help patient to a right side-lying position with head slightly elevated. | [ ] | [ ] | [ ] |
| 6. | Confirm placement of tube in stomach: | | | |
| | a. Attach 60 mL irrigation syringe to tube and inject 10 mL of air while auscultating over epigastrium. Recognize that this may not be reliable index of tube placement if patient has small-bore feeding tube. | [ ] | [ ] | [ ] |
| | b. Aspirate all stomach contents and measure residual. | [ ] | [ ] | [ ] |
| | c. If 100 mL or more than half of last feeding is aspirated, contact physician before proceeding with tube feeding. | [ ] | [ ] | [ ] |
| | d. Reinstill the aspirated gastric contents through tube into stomach. | [ ] | [ ] | [ ] |
| 7. | Prepare correct amount and strength of formula at room temperature. | [ ] | [ ] | [ ] |
| 8. | Connect gavage tubing to gastric tube. | [ ] | [ ] | [ ] |
| 9. | Hang gavage bag on IV pole. | [ ] | [ ] | [ ] |
| 10. | Pour in desired amount of formula according to agency policy. | [ ] | [ ] | [ ] |
| 11. | Connect tubing to infusion pump and set rate. | [ ] | [ ] | [ ] |
| 12. | Check gastric residual every 4 to 6 hours, according to agency policy. Flush tubing with 30 to 60 mL of water. | [ ] | [ ] | [ ] |
| 13. | Have patient remain in high-Fowler's or elevated side-lying position for 30 to 60 minutes. | [ ] | [ ] | [ ] |
| 14. | Wash any reusable equipment with soap and water. Change equipment every 24 hours or according to agency policy. | [ ] | [ ] | [ ] |
| 15. | Wash hands. | [ ] | [ ] | [ ] |
| 16. | Document procedure and observations. | [ ] | [ ] | [ ] |

E = Excels;  S = Satisfactory;  U = Unsatisfactory

COMMENTS:


[ ] Pass  [ ] Fail

Student's Signature_____ Date_____

Instructor's Signature_____ Date _____

© 1992 J.B. Lippincott Company, Fundamentals of Nursing: Human Health and Function

## PROCEDURE 33-3A
# ADMINISTERING TOTAL PARENTERAL NUTRITION (TPN)
## MONITORING TPN THERAPY

|  | E | S | U |
|---|---|---|---|
| 1. Schedule and assist patient with chest x-ray after central catheter insertion. | [ ] | [ ] | [ ] |
| 2. Confirm correct solution is running at ordered rate. Check expiration date of solution. Use infusion controller to monitor and regulate flow rate. | [ ] | [ ] | [ ] |
| 3. Inspect tubing and catheter connection for leaks or kinks. Tape all connections. Change tubing every 24 hours according to agency policy. | [ ] | [ ] | [ ] |
| 4. Inspect insertion site for infiltration, thrombophlebitis, or drainage. If present, notify physician. | [ ] | [ ] | [ ] |
| 5. Monitor vital signs, including temperature, every 4 hours. | [ ] | [ ] | [ ] |
| 6. Assess for symptoms of air embolism: decreased level of consciousness, tachycardia, dyspnea, anxiety, "feeling of impending doom", chest pain, cyanosis, hypotension. If suspected, lay patient on left side with head in Trendelenburg position. | [ ] | [ ] | [ ] |
| 7. Use TPN line only for TPN. | [ ] | [ ] | [ ] |
| 8. Test urine every 6 hours for specific gravity and ketones. | [ ] | [ ] | [ ] |
| 9. Perform test for glucose every 6 hours. Notify physician if abnormal. | [ ] | [ ] | [ ] |
| 10. Monitor laboratory tests of electrolytes, BUN, glucose, as ordered, and report abnormal findings to physician. | [ ] | [ ] | [ ] |
| 11. Maintain accurate record of intake and output to monitor fluid balance. | [ ] | [ ] | [ ] |
| 12. Weigh patient daily and record. | [ ] | [ ] | [ ] |
| 13. Inspect dressing once a shift for drainage and intactness. Change whenever loose or moist and at least every 48 hours. | [ ] | [ ] | [ ] |

E = Excels;  S = Satisfactory;  U = Unsatisfactory

COMMENTS:

[ ] Pass  [ ] Fail

Student's Signature_____ Date_____

Instructor's Signature_____ Date _____

© 1992 J.B. Lippincott Company, Fundamentals of Nursing: Human Health and Function

## PROCEDURE 33-3B
# ADMINISTERING TOTAL PARENTERAL NUTRITION (TPN)
## CHANGING TPN TUBING AND DRESSING

| | E | S | U |
|---|---|---|---|
| 1. Wash hands. | [ ] | [ ] | [ ] |
| 2. Cross-check new hyperalimentation solutions with physician's order.  Check expiration date. | [ ] | [ ] | [ ] |
| 3. Attach sterile tubing and filter to new parenteral hyperalimentation solutions.  Prime tubing as for a conventional IV. | [ ] | [ ] | [ ] |
| 4. Place patient in supine position. | [ ] | [ ] | [ ] |
| 5. Don a mask.  Instruct patient to turn head facing opposite direction of insertion site, and not to cough or talk during dressing change.  Place mask on patient if unable to cooperate. | [ ] | [ ] | [ ] |
| 6. Don gloves. | [ ] | [ ] | [ ] |
| 7. Remove old dressing and discard. | [ ] | [ ] | [ ] |
| 8. Inspect insertion site for redness, drainage, swelling. | [ ] | [ ] | [ ] |
| 9. Remove gloves. | [ ] | [ ] | [ ] |
| 10. Wash hands. | [ ] | [ ] | [ ] |
| 11. Open sterile supplies and place on bedside table. | [ ] | [ ] | [ ] |
| 12. Put on sterile gloves. | [ ] | [ ] | [ ] |
| 13. Cleanse insertion site with gauze soaked in 10% acetone.  Wipe in circular motion, moving from the insertion site outward without touching catheter with acetone. | [ ] | [ ] | [ ] |
| 14. Cleanse site with same circular motion for 2 minutes using povidone-iodine solution (Betadine).  Allow to air dry. | [ ] | [ ] | [ ] |
| 15. Cleanse connection of catheter and tubing with Betadine. | [ ] | [ ] | [ ] |
| 16. Remove Betadine from skin with alcohol, according to agency policy. | [ ] | [ ] | [ ] |
| 17. Apply Betadine ointment to insertion site. | [ ] | [ ] | [ ] |
| 18. Loosen tubing at catheter hub. | [ ] | [ ] | [ ] |
| 19. Ask patient to hold breath and bear down (Valsalva) while quickly disconnecting old tubing and attaching new tubing to catheter hub. | [ ] | [ ] | [ ] |
| 20. Tape all connections. | [ ] | [ ] | [ ] |
| 21. Place transparent, semipermeable dressing over insertion site.  Optional: Paint skin margins with tincture of Benzoin before placing dressing to ensure a tighter seal. | [ ] | [ ] | [ ] |
| 22. Loop and tape tubing next to dressing. | [ ] | [ ] | [ ] |
| 23. Label dressing and tubing with date and name. | [ ] | [ ] | [ ] |

*(continued)*

© 1992 J.B. Lippincott Company, Fundamentals of Nursing:  Human Health and Function

**33-3B:** Administering Total Parenteral Nutrition (TPN)
Changing TPN Tubing And Dressing *(Continued)*

|  | E | S | U |
|---|---|---|---|
| 24. Adjust flow rate per physician's order. | [ ] | [ ] | [ ] |
| 25. Discard used solution and tubing. Remove gloves. | [ ] | [ ] | [ ] |
| 26. Document amount infused on intake and output record. | [ ] | [ ] | [ ] |

E = Excels;  S = Satisfactory;  U = Unsatisfactory

COMMENTS:

[ ] Pass  [ ] Fail

Student's Signature_____ Date_____

Instructor's Signature_____ Date_____

## PROCEDURE 33-3C
# ADMINISTERING TOTAL PARENTERAL NUTRITION (TPN)
### ADMINISTERING INTRALIPIDS

|  | E | S | U |
|---|---|---|---|
| 1. Check solution against physician's order. Inspect solution for separation of emulsion into layers or for froth. Do not use if present. | [ ] | [ ] | [ ] |
| 2. Wash hands. | [ ] | [ ] | [ ] |
| 3. Attach intralipid tubing to bottle. Prime tubing as for a conventional IV. | [ ] | [ ] | [ ] |
| 4. Place 19- or 21-gauge 1 inch needle on distal end of tubing. | [ ] | [ ] | [ ] |
| 5. Identify patient. | [ ] | [ ] | [ ] |
| 6. Identify Y-port on hyperalimentation tubing below in-line filter. | [ ] | [ ] | [ ] |
| 7. Cleanse Y-port with antiseptic swab. Allow to dry. Insert needle into port. Secure with tape. | [ ] | [ ] | [ ] |
| 8. Adjust flow rate to infuse at 1.0 mL/minute for adults and 0.1 mL for children. Infuse at this rate for 30 minutes while monitoring patient and vital signs every 10 minutes. | [ ] | [ ] | [ ] |
| 9. If adverse reactions occur, stop infusion and notify physician. | [ ] | [ ] | [ ] |
| 10. If no adverse reactions occur, adjust flow rate: | | | |
| a. Adults: 500 mL intralipid over 4 to 6 hours. | [ ] | [ ] | [ ] |
| b. Children: up to 1 Gm/Kg over 4 hours. | [ ] | [ ] | [ ] |
| 11. Document procedure according to agency policy. | [ ] | [ ] | [ ] |

E = Excels; S = Satisfactory; U = Unsatisfactory

COMMENTS:

[ ] Pass  [ ] Fail

Student's Signature_____ Date_____

Instructor's Signature_____ Date_____

© 1992 J.B. Lippincott Company, Fundamentals of Nursing: Human Health and Function

# PROCEDURE 34-1
## CHANGING A DRY STERILE DRESSING

|  | | E | S | U |
|---|---|---|---|---|
| 1. | Gather equipment and supplies. | [ ] | [ ] | [ ] |
| 2. | Close patient's door or close curtains around bed. Explain procedure to patient. | [ ] | [ ] | [ ] |
| 3. | Position patient comfortable. Expose only wound area. | [ ] | [ ] | [ ] |
| 4. | Wash hands. | [ ] | [ ] | [ ] |
| 5. | Make a cuff on top of plastic bag and place within easy reach of dressing table. | [ ] | [ ] | [ ] |
| 6. | Put on clean disposable gloves. | [ ] | [ ] | [ ] |
| 7. | Remove dressing from wound and discard into plastic bag. If dressing adheres to wound, pour small amount of sterile saline on wound to loosen dressing. | [ ] | [ ] | [ ] |
| 8. | Remove and dispose of gloves. Wash hands. | [ ] | [ ] | [ ] |
| 9. | Set up sterile supplies. Open sterile towel and hold it by edges. Place on clean, flat surface without contaminating center of towel. Open dressing package(s) by peeling paper down to expose dressing. Let it fall onto sterile field. Open cleansing solution container and applicator packages. Set them at side of sterile field. Optional: Open dressing packages and suture set carefully, allowing the inside of the packaging material to serve as the sterile field. | [ ] | [ ] | [ ] |
| 10. | Don sterile gloves. Grasp applicators at nonabsorbent end and dip into cleansing solution. | [ ] | [ ] | [ ] |
| 11. | Clean drainage from wound with strokes moving from top toward bottom of wound, or from outside toward center. Use each applicator once and discard it. | [ ] | [ ] | [ ] |
| 12. | Dry wound with gauze held by forceps. | [ ] | [ ] | [ ] |
| 13. | Inspect incision for bleeding, inflammation, drainage, and healing. Note any areas of dehiscence. | [ ] | [ ] | [ ] |
| 14. | Apply sterile dressings one at a time over wound. | [ ] | [ ] | [ ] |
| 15. | Secure dressing with tape or Montgomery straps. | [ ] | [ ] | [ ] |
| 16. | Wash hands. | [ ] | [ ] | [ ] |
| 17. | Document procedure and observations. | [ ] | [ ] | [ ] |

E = Excels; S = Satisfactory; U = Unsatisfactory

COMMENTS:


[ ] Pass  [ ] Fail

Student's Signature_____ Date_____

Instructor's Signature_____ Date _____

© 1992 J.B. Lippincott Company, Fundamentals of Nursing: Human Health and Function

## PROCEDURE 34-2
## APPLYING WET-TO-DRY DRESSINGS

| | E | S | U |
|---|---|---|---|
| 1. Gather equipment and supplies. | [ ] | [ ] | [ ] |
| 2. Close patient's door or close curtains around bed. Explain procedure to patient. | [ ] | [ ] | [ ] |
| 3. Position patient comfortably. Expose only wound area. | [ ] | [ ] | [ ] |
| 4. Wash hands. | [ ] | [ ] | [ ] |
| 5. Make a cuff on top of plastic bag and place within easy reach of dressing table. | [ ] | [ ] | [ ] |
| 6. Put on clean disposable gloves. | [ ] | [ ] | [ ] |
| 7. Remove dressing from wound and discard into plastic bag. If desired, use forceps to remove soiled dressing. If dressing adheres to underlying tissue, do not moisten it. Gently remove dressing while assessing patient's discomfort level. | [ ] | [ ] | [ ] |
| 8. Remove and dispose of gloves. Wash hands. | [ ] | [ ] | [ ] |
| 9. Observe dressings for amount and characteristics of drainage. | [ ] | [ ] | [ ] |
| 10. Observe wound for eschar, granulation tissue, or epithelial skin buds. | [ ] | [ ] | [ ] |
| 11. Prepare sterile supplies. Open sterile instruments, sterile basin, solution, and dressings. | [ ] | [ ] | [ ] |
| 12. Place fine-mesh gauze into basin and pour the ordered solution over mesh to saturate. If wound is large, warm the ordered solution. | [ ] | [ ] | [ ] |
| 13. Don sterile gloves. | [ ] | [ ] | [ ] |
| 14. Cleanse wound with antiseptic solution as prescribed or with normal saline, moving from least to most contaminated area. | [ ] | [ ] | [ ] |
| 15. Gently pack moistened gauze into wound. If wound is deep, use forceps or cotton-tipped applicators to press gauze into all wound surfaces. | [ ] | [ ] | [ ] |
| 16. Apply several dry, sterile 4 x 4's over wet gauze. | [ ] | [ ] | [ ] |
| 17. Place ABD pad over 4 x 4's. | [ ] | [ ] | [ ] |
| 18. Remove and dispose of sterile gloves. | [ ] | [ ] | [ ] |
| 19. Secure dressings with tape, Kerlix gauze, or Montgomery ties. | [ ] | [ ] | [ ] |
| 20. Assist patient to comfortable position. | [ ] | [ ] | [ ] |
| 21. Dispose of disposable supplies. Return equipment to storage area. | [ ] | [ ] | [ ] |
| 22. Wash hands. | [ ] | [ ] | [ ] |
| 23. Document procedure and observations. | [ ] | [ ] | [ ] |

E = Excels; S = Satisfactory; U = Unsatisfactory

COMMENTS:

[ ] Pass  [ ] Fail

Student's Signature_____ Date_____

Instructor's Signature_____ Date _____

© 1992 J.B. Lippincott Company, Fundamentals of Nursing: Human Health and Function

## PROCEDURE 34-3
## MAINTAINING A PORTABLE WOUND SUCTION
### HEMOVAC

| | E | S | U |
|---|---|---|---|
| 1. Explain procedure, assist patient to comfortable position, pull curtains or close door. | [ ] | [ ] | [ ] |
| 2. Wash hands. Don clean disposable gloves. | [ ] | [ ] | [ ] |
| 3. Expose Hemovac tubing and container while keeping patient draped. | [ ] | [ ] | [ ] |
| 4. Examine tubing and container for patency and suction seal. | [ ] | [ ] | [ ] |
| 5. Open drainage plug. | [ ] | [ ] | [ ] |
| 6. Pour drainage into a calibrated receptacle without contaminating drainage spout. | [ ] | [ ] | [ ] |
| 7. Reestablish suction by placing reservoir on firm, flat surface. With drainage plug open, compress the unit and reinsert drainage plug. | [ ] | [ ] | [ ] |
| 8. Remove and discard gloves. | [ ] | [ ] | [ ] |
| 9. Return patient to comfortable position. | [ ] | [ ] | [ ] |
| 10. Measure drainage, and record amount, color, and other pertinent information. | [ ] | [ ] | [ ] |

E = Excels; S = Satisfactory; U = Unsatisfactory

COMMENTS:

[ ] Pass [ ] Fail

Student's Signature_____ Date_____

Instructor's Signature_____ Date_____

© 1992 J.B. Lippincott Company, Fundamentals of Nursing: Human Health and Function

114

## PROCEDURE 34-4
## IRRIGATING A WOUND

| | E | S | U |
|---|---|---|---|
| 1. Gather equipment and supplies. | [ ] | [ ] | [ ] |
| 2. Close door or curtains around bed. Explain procedure to patient. | [ ] | [ ] | [ ] |
| 3. Position patient comfortably to allow irrigating solution to flow by gravity across wound and into a collection basin. | [ ] | [ ] | [ ] |
| 4. Expose the wound area only. Place waterproof pad under patient. | [ ] | [ ] | [ ] |
| 5. Wash hands. | [ ] | [ ] | [ ] |
| 6. Don mask, goggles, and gown if needed. | [ ] | [ ] | [ ] |
| 7. Make a cuff on top of plastic bag and place within easy reach of dressing table. | [ ] | [ ] | [ ] |
| 8. Put on clean disposable gloves. | [ ] | [ ] | [ ] |
| 9. Remove dressing from wound and discard into plastic bag. If desired, use forceps to remove soiled dressing. | [ ] | [ ] | [ ] |
| 10. Remove and discard gloves. Wash hands. | [ ] | [ ] | [ ] |
| 11. Observe dressings for amount and characteristics of drainage. Inspect wound. | [ ] | [ ] | [ ] |
| 12. Pour warmed irrigating solution into sterile basin. | [ ] | [ ] | [ ] |
| 13. Open irrigating syringe and place into basin with solution. | [ ] | [ ] | [ ] |
| 14. Place second basin at distal end of wound to catch contaminated irrigating solution. | [ ] | [ ] | [ ] |
| 15. Don sterile gloves. | [ ] | [ ] | [ ] |
| 16. Fill irrigating syringe with solution. Holding syringe tip about an inch above the wound, gently flush all areas of wound. Continue flushing until solution draining into basin is clear. | [ ] | [ ] | [ ] |
| 17. If wound is deep, attach a Robinson catheter to syringe filled with irrigating solution. Gently insert catheter into wound and flush until returning solution is clear. | [ ] | [ ] | [ ] |
| 18. Dry wound edges and surrounding skin with dry gauze dressings. | [ ] | [ ] | [ ] |
| 19. Apply sterile dressing. | [ ] | [ ] | [ ] |
| 20. Remove and discard gloves. | [ ] | [ ] | [ ] |
| 21. Secure dressing with tape or Montgomery straps. | [ ] | [ ] | [ ] |
| 22. Assist patient to comfortable position. | [ ] | [ ] | [ ] |
| 23. Dispose of equipment. Retain remaining bottle of sterile solution for future irrigations. Mark date and time of opening on bottle for reference. | [ ] | [ ] | [ ] |
| 24. Wash hands. | [ ] | [ ] | [ ] |
| 25. Document procedure and observations. | [ ] | [ ] | [ ] |

E = Excels;  S = Satisfactory;  U = Unsatisfactory

COMMENTS:

[ ] Pass  [ ] Fail

Student's Signature_____ Date_____

Instructor's Signature_____ Date _____

© 1992 J.B. Lippincott Company, Fundamentals of Nursing: Human Health and Function

## PROCEDURE 34-5
## APPLYING A COLD PACK

|  | E | S | U |
|---|---|---|---|
| 1. Gather equipment. | [ ] | [ ] | [ ] |
| 2. Prepare ice pack. Fill bag or collar two-thirds full with crushed ice. Expel excess air from bag and secure cap. Commercial pack must be squeezed or kneaded. | [ ] | [ ] | [ ] |
| 3. Place towel or pillowcase over cold pack. | [ ] | [ ] | [ ] |
| 4. Wash hands. | [ ] | [ ] | [ ] |
| 5. Close bed curtains or room door. | [ ] | [ ] | [ ] |
| 6. Assist patient to comfortable position and expose area to be treated. | [ ] | [ ] | [ ] |
| 7. Apply prepared ice pack to area to be treated. Secure with tape or ties if necessary. Cover patient. | [ ] | [ ] | [ ] |
| 8. Monitor condition of skin after 5 minutes. | [ ] | [ ] | [ ] |
| 9. Remove pack after 30 minutes and observe condition of treated skin. | [ ] | [ ] | [ ] |
| 10. Assist patient to comfortable position and dispose of ice or commercial pack. | [ ] | [ ] | [ ] |
| 11. Document procedure and observations. | [ ] | [ ] | [ ] |

E = Excels;  S = Satisfactory;  U = Unsatisfactory

COMMENTS:

[ ] Pass  [ ] Fail

Student's Signature_____ Date_____

Instructor's Signature_____ Date _____

© 1992 J.B. Lippincott Company, Fundamentals of Nursing: Human Health and Function

## PROCEDURE 34-6
## APPLYING AQUATHERMIA PADS

|  | E | S | U |
|---|---|---|---|
| 1. Gather equipment. | [ ] | [ ] | [ ] |
| 2. Close bed curtains or room door. | [ ] | [ ] | [ ] |
| 3. Wash hands. | [ ] | [ ] | [ ] |
| 4. Assist patient to comfortable position and expose area to be treated. | [ ] | [ ] | [ ] |
| 5. Place aquathermia reservoir on bedside stand. Adjust temperature to below 105° F. Plug into electrical outlet. Turn unit on and observe water level in unit. Refill with distilled water, as needed. | [ ] | [ ] | [ ] |
| 6. Cover heating pad with a pillowcase or wrap treatment area with towel. | [ ] | [ ] | [ ] |
| 7. Place pad on affected area and secure with tape if necessary. | [ ] | [ ] | [ ] |
| 8. Monitor skin for erythema five minutes after application. | [ ] | [ ] | [ ] |
| 9. Remove pad after 20 to 30 minutes and store until next treatment. | [ ] | [ ] | [ ] |
| 10. Wait 1 hour before reapplying. | [ ] | [ ] | [ ] |
| 11. Observe treatment area. Question patient to determine comfort level and assess for improved range of motion if used on an extremity. | [ ] | [ ] | [ ] |
| 12. Assist patient to comfortable position. | [ ] | [ ] | [ ] |
| 13. Document procedure and observations. | [ ] | [ ] | [ ] |

E = Excels;  S = Satisfactory;  U = Unsatisfactory

COMMENTS:

[ ] Pass  [ ] Fail

Student's Signature_____ Date_____

Instructor's Signature_____ Date _____

© 1992 J.B. Lippincott Company, Fundamentals of Nursing:  Human Health and Function

# PROCEDURE 37-1A
# COLLECTING URINE SPECIMENS
## STERILE SPECIMEN FROM AN INDWELLING CATHETER

|  | E | S | U |
|---|---|---|---|
| 1. Gather equipment. | [ ] | [ ] | [ ] |
| 2. Explain procedure to patient. | [ ] | [ ] | [ ] |
| 3. Wash hands. Put on clean disposable gloves. | [ ] | [ ] | [ ] |
| 4. Position patient so that catheter is accessible. | [ ] | [ ] | [ ] |
| 5. Cleanse aspiration port of drainage tubing with Betadine swab. | [ ] | [ ] | [ ] |
| 6. Allow at least 2 mL of urine (for culture and sensitivity testing) to collect in tubing by clamping or bending tubing. | [ ] | [ ] | [ ] |
| 7. Insert needle into aspiration port. Draw urine sample into syringe by gentle aspiration. Remove needle. | [ ] | [ ] | [ ] |
| 8. Transfer urine from syringe into a sterile specimen container. | [ ] | [ ] | [ ] |
| 9. Label container. Date and time laboratory requisition. | [ ] | [ ] | [ ] |
| 10. Send specimen to laboratory within 15 minutes or place in specimen refrigerator. Send immediately if specimen is for microbiology testing. | [ ] | [ ] | [ ] |
| 11. Remove and discard gloves. | [ ] | [ ] | [ ] |
| 12. Dispose of all contaminated supplies. Wash hands. | [ ] | [ ] | [ ] |
| 13. Document procedure and observations. | [ ] | [ ] | [ ] |

E = Excels;  S = Satisfactory;  U = Unsatisfactory

COMMENTS:

[ ] Pass  [ ] Fail

Student's Signature_____ Date_____

Instructor's Signature_____ Date _____

© 1992 J.B. Lippincott Company, Fundamentals of Nursing:  Human Health and Function

**118**

## PROCEDURE 37-1B
## COLLECTING URINE SPECIMENS
### COLLECTING MIDSTREAM URINE SPECIMEN FOR A WOMAN

|  | E | S | U |
|---|---|---|---|
| 1. Gather equipment. | [ ] | [ ] | [ ] |
| 2. Instruct patient how to cleanse urinary meatus and obtain urine specimen. | [ ] | [ ] | [ ] |
| 3. Wash hands. | [ ] | [ ] | [ ] |
| 4. Have patient separate labia minora and cleanse perineum with cleansing agent Betadine swab, starting in front of urethral meatus and moving swab toward the rectum. | [ ] | [ ] | [ ] |
| 5. Have patient begin to urinate while continuing to hold labia apart. Allow first urine to flow into toilet. | [ ] | [ ] | [ ] |
| 6. Have patient hold specimen container under urine stream and collect sample. | [ ] | [ ] | [ ] |
| 7. Have patient remove specimen container, release hand from labia, seal container tightly, and finish voiding. | [ ] | [ ] | [ ] |
| 8. Have patient wash hands. | [ ] | [ ] | [ ] |
| 9. Don clean disposable gloves to receive specimen container from patient. Cleanse and rinse outer surface of container with disinfectant. Remove and discard gloves. | [ ] | [ ] | [ ] |
| 10. Label container. Date and time laboratory requisition. | [ ] | [ ] | [ ] |
| 11. Send specimen to laboratory within 15 minutes or place in specimen refrigerator. Send immediately if specimen is for microbiology testing. | [ ] | [ ] | [ ] |
| 12. Dispose of all contaminated supplies. Wash hands. | [ ] | [ ] | [ ] |
| 13. Document procedure and observations. | [ ] | [ ] | [ ] |

E = Excels; S = Satisfactory; U = Unsatisfactory

COMMENTS:

[ ] Pass  [ ] Fail

Student's Signature_____ Date_____

Instructor's Signature_____ Date _____

© 1992 J.B. Lippincott Company, Fundamentals of Nursing: Human Health and Function

# PROCEDURE 37-1C
## COLLECTING URINE SPECIMENS
### COLLECTING MIDSTREAM URINE SPECIMEN FOR A MAN

|  | E | S | U |
|---|---|---|---|
| 1. Gather equipment. | [ ] | [ ] | [ ] |
| 2. Instruct patient how to cleanse urinary meatus and obtain urine specimen. | [ ] | [ ] | [ ] |
| 3. Wash hands. | [ ] | [ ] | [ ] |
| 4. Have patient cleanse end of penis with cleansing agent Betadine swab. If uncircumcised, instruct him to retract foreskin to expose urinary meatus before cleansing and throughout specimen collection. | [ ] | [ ] | [ ] |
| 5. Have patient begin to urinate allowing first urine to flow into toilet. | [ ] | [ ] | [ ] |
| 6. Have patient hold specimen container under urine stream and collect sample. | [ ] | [ ] | [ ] |
| 7. Have patient remove specimen container, seal container tightly, and finish voiding. | [ ] | [ ] | [ ] |
| 8. Have patient wash hands. | [ ] | [ ] | [ ] |
| 9. Don clean disposable gloves to receive specimen container from patient. Cleanse and rinse outer surface of container with disinfectant. Remove and discard gloves. | [ ] | [ ] | [ ] |
| 10. Label container. Date and time laboratory requisition. | [ ] | [ ] | [ ] |
| 11. Send specimen to laboratory within 15 minutes or place in specimen refrigerator. Send immediately if specimen is for microbiology testing. | [ ] | [ ] | [ ] |
| 12. Dispose of all contaminated supplies. Wash hands. | [ ] | [ ] | [ ] |
| 13. Document procedure and observations. | [ ] | [ ] | [ ] |

E = Excels;  S = Satisfactory;  U = Unsatisfactory

COMMENTS:

[ ] Pass  [ ] Fail

Student's Signature_____ Date_____

Instructor's Signature_____ Date _____

© 1992 J.B. Lippincott Company, Fundamentals of Nursing: Human Health and Function

## PROCEDURE 37-1D
## COLLECTING URINE SPECIMENS
## FROM CHILD WITHOUT URINARY CONTROL

|  | E | S | U |
|---|---|---|---|
| 1. Wash hands. | [ ] | [ ] | [ ] |
| 2. Explain procedure to parents of child if present. | [ ] | [ ] | [ ] |
| 3. Position child gently on back. Put on clean disposable gloves Remove diaper. | [ ] | [ ] | [ ] |
| 4. Clean perineal-genital area gently with soap and water, followed by Betadine antiseptic. | [ ] | [ ] | [ ] |
| 5. For a girl: Separate labia and cleanse from front of urethral meatus toward rectum. Rinse with sterile water and dry with cotton balls. | [ ] | [ ] | [ ] |
| 6. For a boy: Cleanse penis and scrotum. If uncircumcised, retract foreskin and cleanse. Rinse with sterile water and dry with gauze or cotton balls. | [ ] | [ ] | [ ] |
| 7. Remove paper backing from adhesive of collection bag. | [ ] | [ ] | [ ] |
| 8. Spread child's legs apart widely. | [ ] | [ ] | [ ] |
| 9. Apply collection bag over child's perineum, covering penis and scrotum on boy, and urinary meatus and vagina of girl. Press adhesive to secure, starting at perineum and working outward. | [ ] | [ ] | [ ] |
| 10. Place a diaper on child loosely. | [ ] | [ ] | [ ] |
| 11. Remove gloves and wash hands. | [ ] | [ ] | [ ] |
| 12. Check the collector for urine every 15 minutes. | [ ] | [ ] | [ ] |
| 13. When urine specimen is obtained, glove again, and gently remove collection bag from skin and empty urine into specimen container. | [ ] | [ ] | [ ] |
| 14. Tighten lid and cleanse outside of container if contaminated with urine. Remove and discard gloves. | [ ] | [ ] | [ ] |
| 15. Label the container. Date and time laboratory requisition. | [ ] | [ ] | [ ] |
| 16. Send specimen to laboratory within 15 minutes or place in specimen refrigerator. Send immediately if specimen is for microbiology testing. | [ ] | [ ] | [ ] |
| 17. Dispose of all contaminated supplies. Wash hands. | [ ] | [ ] | [ ] |
| 18. Document that specimen was collected and sent. | [ ] | [ ] | [ ] |

E = Excels;  S = Satisfactory;  U = Unsatisfactory

COMMENTS:


[ ] Pass  [ ] Fail

Student's Signature_____ Date_____

Instructor's Signature_____ Date _____

© 1992 J.B. Lippincott Company, Fundamentals of Nursing: Human Health and Function

## PROCEDURE 37-2
## TESTING SPECIFIC GRAVITY OF URINE

|  | E | S | U |
|---|---|---|---|
| 1. Gather equipment. | [ ] | [ ] | [ ] |
| 2. Wash hands. Put on clean disposable gloves. | [ ] | [ ] | [ ] |
| 3. Pour urine into glass cylinder until it is one-half to three-quarters full. | [ ] | [ ] | [ ] |
| 4. Place urometer into cylinder. Gently spin stem of urometer. | [ ] | [ ] | [ ] |
| 5. Place cylinder on flat surface at eye level. When twirling stops, read where the urine level meets the calibrated urometer at the base of the meniscus. | [ ] | [ ] | [ ] |
| 6. Discard urine, wash equipment with soap and water, allow to air dry. | [ ] | [ ] | [ ] |
| 7. Remove and discard gloves. Wash hands. | [ ] | [ ] | [ ] |
| 8. Document findings. | [ ] | [ ] | [ ] |

E = Excels;  S = Satisfactory;  U = Unsatisfactory

COMMENTS:

[ ] Pass  [ ] Fail

Student's Signature_____ Date_____

Instructor's Signature_____ Date _____

© 1992 J.B. Lippincott Company, Fundamentals of Nursing: Human Health and Function

122

## PROCEDURE 37-3
## APPLYING A CONDOM CATHETER

|  | E | S | U |
|---|---|---|---|
| 1. Gather equipment. | [ ] | [ ] | [ ] |
| 2. Close room door or bedside curtain. Explain procedure to patient. | [ ] | [ ] | [ ] |
| 3. Wash hands. | [ ] | [ ] | [ ] |
| 4. Assist patient to supine position with genitalia exposed. | [ ] | [ ] | [ ] |
| 5. Put on clean disposable gloves. Wash genitals with soap and water. Towel dry. | [ ] | [ ] | [ ] |
| 6. Trim or shave excess pubic hair from base of penis, if necessary. | [ ] | [ ] | [ ] |
| 7. Apply thin film of skin protector on penis shaft. Allow to dry for 30 seconds. | [ ] | [ ] | [ ] |
| 8. Peel paper backing from both sides of adhesive line and wrap spirally around penis shaft. | [ ] | [ ] | [ ] |
| 9. Place funnel end of pre-rolled condom against glans of penis. Unroll sheath the length of the penis, over the adhesive liner. | [ ] | [ ] | [ ] |
| 10. Attach funnel end of condom to collection system. Secure system below level of condom, avoiding kinks or loops in tubing. | [ ] | [ ] | [ ] |
| 11. Discard used supplies. Remove and discard gloves. Wash hands. | [ ] | [ ] | [ ] |
| 12. Observe penis 15 to 30 minutes after application of condom for swelling or changes in skin color. | [ ] | [ ] | [ ] |
| 13. Document procedure and observations. | [ ] | [ ] | [ ] |

E = Excels;  S = Satisfactory;  U = Unsatisfactory

COMMENTS:

[ ] Pass  [ ] Fail

Student's Signature_____ Date_____

Instructor's Signature_____ Date_____

© 1992 J.B. Lippincott Company, Fundamentals of Nursing: Human Health and Function

## PROCEDURE 37-4A
# INSERTING A STRAIGHT OR INDWELLING CATHETER
## WOMAN

|  | E | S | U |
|---|---|---|---|
| 1. Gather equipment. | [ ] | [ ] | [ ] |
| 2. Explain procedure and rationale to patient. | [ ] | [ ] | [ ] |
| 3. Provide patient with opportunity to perform personal perineal hygiene.  Assist patient as necessary. | [ ] | [ ] | [ ] |
| 4. Wash hands. | [ ] | [ ] | [ ] |
| 5. Position in dorsal recumbent position.  Externally rotate thighs.  Side-lying is alternate position. | [ ] | [ ] | [ ] |
| 6. Drape legs to midthigh with bath blanket. | [ ] | [ ] | [ ] |
| 7. Set up light source. | [ ] | [ ] | [ ] |
| 8. Open catheterization tray. | [ ] | [ ] | [ ] |
| 9. Put on sterile gloves. | [ ] | [ ] | [ ] |
| 10. Slide sterile drape under patient's buttocks, protecting gloved hands with corners of drape or ask patient to lift hips so drape can be positioned. | [ ] | [ ] | [ ] |
| 11. Open sterile lubricant and lubricate catheter tip. | [ ] | [ ] | [ ] |
| 12. Open cleansing solution and pour over half of the sterile cotton balls.  Open sterile specimen container.  Inflate balloon with pre-filled syringe to check for defective balloon.  Aspirate fluid back into syringe and leave attached. | [ ] | [ ] | [ ] |
| 13. Place nondominant hand on labia minora and gently spread to expose urinary meatus.  Visualize exact location of meatus.  During cleansing and catheter insertion, do not allow labia to close over meatus until after catheter is inserted. | [ ] | [ ] | [ ] |
| 14. Using sterile hand, pick up antiseptic solution saturated cotton ball with sterile forceps. | [ ] | [ ] | [ ] |
| 15. Cleanse urinary meatus with one downward stroke.  Discard cotton ball.  Repeat this step three or four times. | [ ] | [ ] | [ ] |
| 16. Use forceps and two dry cotton balls to dry meatus. | [ ] | [ ] | [ ] |
| 17. With sterile hand, pick up catheter approximately three inches from tip and dip into sterile lubricant.  Place distal catheter end into sterile basin. | [ ] | [ ] | [ ] |
| 18. Gently insert catheter into urethra approximately 2 inches until urine begins to drain. | [ ] | [ ] | [ ] |
| 19. Insert catheter an additional 1 inch or 2.5 cm.  If catheter enters vagina by mistake, leave it there as a landmark.  Insert second catheter into meatus. | [ ] | [ ] | [ ] |
| 20. Obtain urine specimen in sterile container, if ordered. | [ ] | [ ] | [ ] |
| 21. If using straight catheter:  Allow bladder to empty, then remove straight catheter. | [ ] | [ ] | [ ] |

*(continued)*

© 1992 J.B. Lippincott Company, Fundamentals of Nursing:  Human Health and Function

**37-4A:  Inserting A Straight Or Indwelling Catheter
Woman   *(Continued)*

|                                                                                                                        | E | S | U |
|------------------------------------------------------------------------------------------------------------------------|---|---|---|
| 22. If using indwelling catheter: Inflate the retention balloon with the prefilled syringe.                            |   |   |   |
| 23. Check to assure placement by gently pulling on catheter.                                                           | [ ] | [ ] | [ ] |
| 24. Connect distal end of catheter to drainage bag.                                                                    | [ ] | [ ] | [ ] |
| 25. Tape catheter securely with 1-inch tape to inner thigh with enough give so it will not pull when moving the legs.  | [ ] | [ ] | [ ] |
| 26. Attach drainage bag to bed frame, assuring that tubing does not fall into dependent loops or that siderails do not interfere with drainage system. | [ ] | [ ] | [ ] |
| 27. Remove and discard gloves.  Wash hands.                                                                            | [ ] | [ ] | [ ] |
| 28. Record time procedure was complete, size of catheter inserted, amount and color of urine and any adverse patient responses. | [ ] | [ ] | [ ] |

E = Excels;  S = Satisfactory;  U = Unsatisfactory

COMMENTS:

[ ] Pass  [ ] Fail

Student's Signature_____ Date_____

Instructor's Signature_____ Date _____

© 1992 J.B. Lippincott Company, Fundamentals of Nursing:  Human Health and Function

## PROCEDURE 37-4B
# INSERTING A STRAIGHT OR INDWELLING CATHETER
## MAN

| | E | S | U |
|---|---|---|---|
| 1. Gather equipment. | [ ] | [ ] | [ ] |
| 2. Explain procedure and rationale to patient. | [ ] | [ ] | [ ] |
| 3. Provide patient with opportunity to perform personal penile hygiene. Assist patient as necessary. | [ ] | [ ] | [ ] |
| 4. Wash hands. | [ ] | [ ] | [ ] |
| 5. Position in supine position. | [ ] | [ ] | [ ] |
| 6. Drape legs to midthigh with bath blanket. | [ ] | [ ] | [ ] |
| 7. Set up light source. | [ ] | [ ] | [ ] |
| 8. Open catheterization tray. | [ ] | [ ] | [ ] |
| 9. Put on sterile gloves. Open sterile lubricant and lubricate catheter tip. Open cleansing solution and pour over half of the sterile cotton balls. Open sterile specimen container. Inflate balloon with prefilled syringe to check for defective balloon. Aspirate fluid back into syringe and leave attached. | [ ] | [ ] | [ ] |
| 10. Place fenestrated drape over patient's genitalia. | [ ] | [ ] | [ ] |
| 11. With nondominant hand, hold penis at a 90 degree angle to his body. If uncircumcised, pull down foreskin with this hand to visualize urethral meatus. | [ ] | [ ] | [ ] |
| 12. Using sterile hand, pick up antiseptic solution saturated cotton ball with sterile forceps. | [ ] | [ ] | [ ] |
| 13. Cleanse urinary meatus with one downward stroke or use circular motion from meatus to base of penis. Discard cotton ball. Repeat this step three or four times. | [ ] | [ ] | [ ] |
| 14. Use forceps to pick up one dry cotton ball to dry meatus. | [ ] | [ ] | [ ] |
| 15. With sterile hand, pick up catheter approximately three inches from tip and dip into sterile lubricant. Place distal catheter end into sterile basin. | [ ] | [ ] | [ ] |
| 16. Gently insert catheter into urethra approximately 8 inches until urine begins to drain. | [ ] | [ ] | [ ] |
| 17. Insert catheter an additional 1 inch or 2.5 cm. | [ ] | [ ] | [ ] |
| 18. Obtain urine specimen in sterile container, if ordered. | [ ] | [ ] | [ ] |
| 19. If using straight catheter: Allow bladder to empty, then remove straight catheter. | [ ] | [ ] | [ ] |
| 20. If using indwelling catheter: Inflate the retention balloon with the prefilled syringe. | [ ] | [ ] | [ ] |
| 21. Check to assure placement by gently pulling on catheter. | [ ] | [ ] | [ ] |
| 22. Connect distal end of catheter to drainage bag. | [ ] | [ ] | [ ] |
| 23. Tape catheter securely with 1-inch tape to abdomen to prevent trauma to penoscrotal angle. | [ ] | [ ] | [ ] |
| 24. In uncircumcised male, gently replace foreskin over glans. | [ ] | [ ] | [ ] |

*(continued)*

© 1992 J.B. Lippincott Company, Fundamentals of Nursing: Human Health and Function

## 37-4B: Inserting A Straight Or Indwelling Catheter - Man *(Continued)*

|  | E | S | U |
|---|---|---|---|
| 25. Attach drainage bag to bed frame, assuring that tubing does not fall into dependent loops or that siderails do not interfere with drainage system. | [ ] | [ ] | [ ] |
| 26. Remove and discard gloves.  Wash hands. | [ ] | [ ] | [ ] |
| 27. Record time procedure was complete, size of catheter inserted, amount and color of urine and any adverse patient responses. | [ ] | [ ] | [ ] |

E = Excels;  S = Satisfactory;  U = Unsatisfactory

COMMENTS:

[ ] Pass  [ ] Fail

Student's Signature_____ Date_____

Instructor's Signature_____ Date _____

© 1992 J.B. Lippincott Company, Fundamentals of Nursing:  Human Health and Function

## PROCEDURE 37-4C
## REMOVING AN INDWELLING CATHETER

|  | E | S | U |
|---|---|---|---|
| 1. Wash hands. | [ ] | [ ] | [ ] |
| 2. Don clean disposable gloves. | [ ] | [ ] | [ ] |
| 3. Clamp catheter (optional). | [ ] | [ ] | [ ] |
| 4. Insert hub of syringe into balloon inflation tube of catheter and draw out all liquid. | [ ] | [ ] | [ ] |
| 5. Ask patient to breathe in and out deeply. Gently remove catheter as patient exhales. | [ ] | [ ] | [ ] |
| 6. Assist patient to cleanse and dry genitals. | [ ] | [ ] | [ ] |
| 7. Measure and document urine in drainage bag and time of catheter removal. | [ ] | [ ] | [ ] |
| 8. Wash hands. | [ ] | [ ] | [ ] |

E = Excels;  S = Satisfactory;  U = Unsatisfactory

COMMENTS:

[ ] Pass  [ ] Fail

Student's Signature_____ Date_____

Instructor's Signature_____ Date _____

© 1992 J.B. Lippincott Company, Fundamentals of Nursing: Human Health and Function

# PROCEDURE 37-5
## PERFORMING CONTINUOUS BLADDER IRRIGATION

|  | E | S | U |
|---|---|---|---|
| 1. Gather equipment. | [ ] | [ ] | [ ] |
| 2. Wash hands. | [ ] | [ ] | [ ] |
| 3. Close room door or pull bed curtains, and drape patient with bath blanket. | [ ] | [ ] | [ ] |
| 4. Explain procedure to patient. | [ ] | [ ] | [ ] |
| 5. Don clean disposable gloves. Empty and record amount of urine in drainage bag. Remove and dispose of soiled gloves. | [ ] | [ ] | [ ] |
| 6. Wash hands. | [ ] | [ ] | [ ] |
| 7. Connect sterile tubing to irrigation solution using aseptic technique. Hang solution container on IV pole. | [ ] | [ ] | [ ] |
| 8. Flush fluid through tubing, maintaining sterility of distal end. | [ ] | [ ] | [ ] |
| 9. Connect input port of three-way catheter to irrigating tubing. | [ ] | [ ] | [ ] |
| 10. Open flow clamp on irrigation tubing and adjust drip rate as ordered. | [ ] | [ ] | [ ] |
| 11. Tape catheter securely with 1 inch tape to thigh for a woman and to abdomen for a man. | [ ] | [ ] | [ ] |
| 12. Assist patient to comfortable position. | [ ] | [ ] | [ ] |
| 13. Inspect drainage for color, clarity, and amount. | [ ] | [ ] | [ ] |
| 14. Wash hands. | [ ] | [ ] | [ ] |
| 15. Document procedure and observations. | [ ] | [ ] | [ ] |
| 16. Measure and record intake and output every two hours or according to agency protocol. | [ ] | [ ] | [ ] |
| 17. Calculate actual urine output by subtracting amount of irrigation infused from the amount of drainage obtained. | [ ] | [ ] | [ ] |

E = Excels;  S = Satisfactory;  U = Unsatisfactory

COMMENTS:

[ ] Pass  [ ] Fail

Student's Signature_____ Date_____

Instructor's Signature_____ Date _____

© 1992 J.B. Lippincott Company, Fundamentals of Nursing: Human Health and Function

## PROCEDURE 38-1A
## ASSESSING STOOL FOR OCCULT BLOOD
### HEMOCCULT SLIDE TEST

|  | E | S | U |
|---|---|---|---|
| 1. Ask patient to void before collecting stool specimen. | [ ] | [ ] | [ ] |
| 2. Assist patient onto bedpan, commode, or to bathroom. Provide privacy and leave call bell within reach. | [ ] | [ ] | [ ] |
| 3. When patient has passed stool and is clean and comfortable, don disposable gloves and obtain small amount of stool with tongue blade or wooden applicator. | [ ] | [ ] | [ ] |
| 4. Open flap of slide and apply a very thin smear of stool onto first window. | [ ] | [ ] | [ ] |
| 5. Using second applicator, obtain a second sample from a different area of stool. Smear thinly on second window of slide. | [ ] | [ ] | [ ] |
| 6. Close slide cover. Open flap on reverse side and apply two drops of hemo-occult developing solution onto each window. | [ ] | [ ] | [ ] |
| 7. Wait 30 to 60 seconds. Read test results. | [ ] | [ ] | [ ] |
| 8. Remove and discard gloves. Wash hands and document findings. | [ ] | [ ] | [ ] |

E = Excels;  S = Satisfactory;  U = Unsatisfactory

COMMENTS:

[ ] Pass  [ ] Fail

Student's Signature_____ Date_____

Instructor's Signature_____ Date _____

© 1992 J.B. Lippincott Company, Fundamentals of Nursing: Human Health and Function

## PROCEDURE 38-1B
## ASSESSING STOOL FOR OCCULT BLOOD
### HEMATEST TABLETS

|  | E | S | U |
|---|---|---|---|
| 1. Ask patient to void before collecting stool specimen. | [ ] | [ ] | [ ] |
| 2. Assist patient onto bedpan, commode, or to bathroom. Provide privacy and leave call bell within reach. | [ ] | [ ] | [ ] |
| 3. When patient has passed stool and is clean and comfortable, don disposable gloves and obtain small amount of stool with tongue blade or wooden applicator. | [ ] | [ ] | [ ] |
| 4. Apply small smear of stool onto guaiac filter paper. | [ ] | [ ] | [ ] |
| 5. Place hematest tablet on stool sample. | [ ] | [ ] | [ ] |
| 6. Apply two to three drops of water onto hematest tablet. Hold paper so water runs onto guaiac paper. | [ ] | [ ] | [ ] |
| 7. Read test results within 2 minutes by observing color of guaiac paper. | [ ] | [ ] | [ ] |
| 8. Remove and discard gloves. Wash hands and document findings. | [ ] | [ ] | [ ] |

E = Excels;  S = Satisfactory;  U = Unsatisfactory

COMMENTS:

[ ] Pass  [ ] Fail

Student's Signature_____  Date_____

Instructor's Signature_____  Date _____

© 1992 J.B. Lippincott Company, Fundamentals of Nursing:  Human Health and Function

# PROCEDURE 38-2
## ADMINISTERING AN ENEMA
### LARGE VOLUME

|  | E | S | U |
|---|---|---|---|
| 1. Gather equipment. Wash hands. | [ ] | [ ] | [ ] |
| 2. Provide patient with privacy by closing curtains or door. | [ ] | [ ] | [ ] |
| 3. Have patient lie on left side (Sim's position) with right knee flexed. Children and adults with poor sphincter control are placed in dorsal recumbent position on a bedpan. | [ ] | [ ] | [ ] |
| 4. Place waterproof towel under patient's buttocks. | [ ] | [ ] | [ ] |
| 5. Cover patient with bath blanket, exposing only the rectum. | [ ] | [ ] | [ ] |
| 6. Put on disposable gloves. | [ ] | [ ] | [ ] |
| 7. Fill enema bag with 750 to 1000 mL lukewarm solution at 105 to 110 degrees F. For a child, 500 mL or less at 100 degrees F. Check temperature of solution with bath thermometer or by pouring small amount over inner wrist. | [ ] | [ ] | [ ] |
| 8. Open clamp on tubing and flush solution to remove air. Reclamp tubing. | [ ] | [ ] | [ ] |
| 9. Lubricate 2 to 3 inches of tip of rectal tube with water-soluble lubricant. | [ ] | [ ] | [ ] |
| 10. Separate buttocks to visualize anus. Observe for external hemorrhoids, ask patient to take slow, deep breath, and gently insert rectal tube directing tip toward the umbilicus (adult, 3 to 4 inches; child, 2 to 3 inches; infant, 1 to 1.5 inches). | [ ] | [ ] | [ ] |
| 11. Continue holding tube in rectum. With other hand open clamp and allow solution to slowly enter patient. Raise container 18 inches above the anus, allowing solution to flow in slowly over a period of 5 to 10 minutes. If patient complains of cramping or pain, have patient breathe deeply and lower bag until sensation stops. | [ ] | [ ] | [ ] |
| 12. Reclamp tubing when all solution has infused. | [ ] | [ ] | [ ] |
| 13. Remove tube gently and have patient squeeze buttocks together firmly for several minutes until urge to defecate caused by tube removal has passed. | [ ] | [ ] | [ ] |
| 14. Have patient retain solution as long as possible. | [ ] | [ ] | [ ] |
| 15. Assist patient to bathroom, commode, or bedpan. Place call bell within reach. Provide privacy until all solution has been expelled. | [ ] | [ ] | [ ] |
| 16. Visually inspect character of the feces and solution. | [ ] | [ ] | [ ] |
| 17. Assist patient to position of comfort. | [ ] | [ ] | [ ] |

*(continued)*

© 1992 J.B. Lippincott Company, Fundamentals of Nursing: Human Health and Function

**38-2: Administering An Enema - Large Volume** *(Continued)*

|  | E | S | U |
|---|---|---|---|
| 18. Assist with cleansing of patient as needed. Provide materials for patient to wash hands. Open windows or provide air freshener if needed. Clean and dispose of equipment as necessary. Remove gloves and wash hands. | [ ] | [ ] | [ ] |
| 19. Document procedure and observations. | [ ] | [ ] | [ ] |

E = Excels;   S = Satisfactory;   U = Unsatisfactory

COMMENTS:

[ ] Pass  [ ] Fail

Student's Signature_____ Date_____

Instructor's Signature_____ Date _____

© 1992 J.B. Lippincott Company, Fundamentals of Nursing: Human Health and Function

# PROCEDURE 38-2B
## ADMINISTERING AN ENEMA
### SMALL VOLUME

|  | E | S | U |
|---|---|---|---|
| 1. Gather equipment. Wash hands. | [ ] | [ ] | [ ] |
| 2. Provide patient with privacy by closing curtains or door. | [ ] | [ ] | [ ] |
| 3. Have patient lie on left side (Sim's position) with right knee flexed. Children and adults with poor sphincter control are placed in dorsal recumbent position on a bedpan. | [ ] | [ ] | [ ] |
| 4. Place waterproof towel under patient's buttocks. | [ ] | [ ] | [ ] |
| 5. Cover patient with bath blanket, exposing only the rectum. | [ ] | [ ] | [ ] |
| 6. Put on disposable gloves. | [ ] | [ ] | [ ] |
| 7. Remove protective cap from prelubricated catheter tip. You may add more lubricant if necessary. | [ ] | [ ] | [ ] |
| 8. Separate buttocks to visualize anus. Observe for hemorrhoids and gently insert rectal tip into rectum. Advance 3 to 4 inches in an adult, directing tip toward umbilicus. | [ ] | [ ] | [ ] |
| 9. Squeeze bottle to empty contents into rectum and colon (approximately 240 mL solution). | [ ] | [ ] | [ ] |
| 10. Maintain pressure on bottle until withdrawn from rectum. | [ ] | [ ] | [ ] |
| 11. Remove tube gently and have patient squeeze buttocks together firmly for several minutes until urge to defecate caused by tube removal has passed. | [ ] | [ ] | [ ] |
| 12. Have patient retain solution as long as possible. | [ ] | [ ] | [ ] |
| 13. Assist patient to bathroom, commode, or bedpan. Place call bell within reach. Provide privacy until all solution has been expelled. | [ ] | [ ] | [ ] |
| 14. Visually inspect character of the feces and solution. | [ ] | [ ] | [ ] |
| 15. Assist patient to position of comfort. | [ ] | [ ] | [ ] |
| 16. Assist with cleansing of patient as needed. Provide materials for patient to wash hands. Open windows or provide air freshener if needed. Clean and dispose of equipment as necessary. Remove gloves and wash hands. | [ ] | [ ] | [ ] |
| 17. Document procedure and observations. | [ ] | [ ] | [ ] |

E = Excels;  S = Satisfactory;  U = Unsatisfactory

COMMENTS:

[ ] Pass  [ ] Fail

Student's Signature_____ Date_____

Instructor's Signature_____ Date _____

© 1992 J.B. Lippincott Company, Fundamentals of Nursing: Human Health and Function

## PROCEDURE 38-3
## INSERTING A NASOGASTRIC TUBE

| | E | S | U |
|---|---|---|---|
| 1. Gather equipment. | [ ] | [ ] | [ ] |
| 2. Identify patient and explain procedure. | [ ] | [ ] | [ ] |
| 3. Provide privacy by closing curtains or door. | [ ] | [ ] | [ ] |
| 4. Raise bed to high-Fowler's position, cover chest with towel, and place emesis basin nearby. | [ ] | [ ] | [ ] |
| 5. Wash hands. | [ ] | [ ] | [ ] |
| 6. Determine length of tubing to be inserted by measuring nasogastric tube from tip of ear lobe to tip of nose, then to tip of xiphoid process. Mark tubing with adhesive tape or note striped markings already on tube. | [ ] | [ ] | [ ] |
| 7. Lubricate tip of tube with water soluble lubricant. | [ ] | [ ] | [ ] |
| 8. Gently insert tube into nostril. Advance toward posterior pharynx by aiming back and toward ear. | [ ] | [ ] | [ ] |
| 9. Have patient tilt head forward and encourage patient to drink water slowly. Advance tube without using force as patient swallows. Advance tube until desired insertion length is reached. | [ ] | [ ] | [ ] |
| 10. Assess placement of tube: a. Aspirate gastric content with 20 to 50 mL syringe. | [ ] | [ ] | [ ] |
| b. Auscultate over epigastrium while injecting 10 to 20 mL air into nasogastric tube. | [ ] | [ ] | [ ] |
| 11. If placement in stomach is not verified, advance tube 5 cm and repeat assessment in step 10. | [ ] | [ ] | [ ] |
| 12. Secure tube by taping to bridge of patient's nose. Anchor tubing to patient's gown. | [ ] | [ ] | [ ] |
| 13. Clamp end of tubing or attach to suction, as ordered by physician. | [ ] | [ ] | [ ] |
| 14. Wash hands, provide for patient's comfort, and clean up equipment. | [ ] | [ ] | [ ] |
| 15. Establish and document a nursing plan for daily care of nasogastric tube: a. Inspecting nostril for irritation. b. Cleansing nare around tube. c. Changing adhesive as required to prevent skin irritation or pressure sores on nare from tube. | [ ] | [ ] | [ ] |

*(continued)*

© 1992 J.B. Lippincott Company, Fundamentals of Nursing: Human Health and Function

**38-3: Inserting A Nasogastric Tube** *(Continued)*

|  | E | S | U |
|---|---|---|---|

      **d. Increase frequency of oral care since patients with nasogastric tubes often mouth breathe and may be NPO.**

**16. Document procedure and observations.**     [ ]  [ ]  [ ]

**E = Excels; S = Satisfactory; U = Unsatisfactory**

**COMMENTS:**

**[ ] Pass [ ] Fail**

**Student's Signature**_____ **Date**_____

**Instructor's Signature**_____ **Date** _____

© 1992 J.B. Lippincott Company, Fundamentals of Nursing: Human Health and Function

## PROCEDURE 38-4
## APPLYING A FECAL OSTOMY POUCH

| | E | S | U |
|---|---|---|---|
| 1. Gather equipment.  Wash hands. | [ ] | [ ] | [ ] |
| 2. Close curtains around bed or close door. | [ ] | [ ] | [ ] |
| 3. Explain procedure to patient. | [ ] | [ ] | [ ] |
| 4. Don disposable gloves.  Gently remove old appliance. If disposable, discard.  If reusable, set aside for washing. | [ ] | [ ] | [ ] |
| 5. Wash skin thoroughly around stoma with skin cleanser or soap and water. | [ ] | [ ] | [ ] |
| 6. Rinse skin thoroughly and blot dry. | [ ] | [ ] | [ ] |
| 7. Observe condition of peristomal skin, the stoma, and the sutures.  Teach patient to make these observations daily. | [ ] | [ ] | [ ] |
| 8. Prepare clean pouch.  Measure stoma and trace circle 1/8-inch larger than stoma on adhesive paper backing.  Cut stoma pattern. | [ ] | [ ] | [ ] |
| 9. Prepare skin barrier.  Measure stoma and cut hole in barrier the same size as stoma.  Be sure edges are rounded. | [ ] | [ ] | [ ] |
| 10. If stoma located in abdominal crease or skin is irregular, use paste barrier to fill the irregularity. | [ ] | [ ] | [ ] |
| 11. Remove paper backing from pouch adhesive faceplate. Center and apply the nonadhesive side of barrier over skin. | [ ] | [ ] | [ ] |
| 12. Remove paper backing from barrier.  Center barrier/pouch unit over the stoma and apply, smoothing out from the center. | [ ] | [ ] | [ ] |
| 13. "Picture frame" the faceplate with hypo-allergenic tape. | [ ] | [ ] | [ ] |
| 14. Fold over bottom edge of pouch and clamp. | [ ] | [ ] | [ ] |
| 15. Dispose of old appliance.  Remove and discard gloves. Clean and store any reusable supplies. | [ ] | [ ] | [ ] |
| 16. Wash hands. | [ ] | [ ] | [ ] |
| 17. Document noted observations. | [ ] | [ ] | [ ] |

E = Excels;  S = Satisfactory;  U = Unsatisfactory

COMMENTS:

[ ] Pass  [ ] Fail

Student's Signature_____ Date_____

Instructor's Signature_____ Date _____

© 1992 J.B. Lippincott Company, Fundamentals of Nursing:  Human Health and Function

## PROCEDURE 38-5
## IRRIGATING A COLOSTOMY

|  | E | S | U |
|---|---|---|---|
| 1. Gather equipment. Wash hands. | [ ] | [ ] | [ ] |
| 2. Prepare patient by explaining procedure. | [ ] | [ ] | [ ] |
| 3. Plan appropriate time for procedure. | [ ] | [ ] | [ ] |
| 4. Assist patient to comfortable position. If ambulatory, have patient sit on toilet. If on bedrest, have patient lie on side. | [ ] | [ ] | [ ] |
| 5. Close bathroom door or bed curtains. | [ ] | [ ] | [ ] |
| 6. Don gloves. | [ ] | [ ] | [ ] |
| 7. Remove and dispose of used pouch. Clean stoma and surrounding skin with warm water and soft cloth. | [ ] | [ ] | [ ] |
| 8. Apply irrigating sleeve. Place sleeve into toilet. If done in bed, place in bedpan. | [ ] | [ ] | [ ] |
| 9. Fill container with 500 to 1000 mL warm water (105 to 110 degrees F.). | [ ] | [ ] | [ ] |
| 10. Connect cone to irrigating tube and run water through entire length of tubing. | [ ] | [ ] | [ ] |
| 11. Apply water-soluble lubricant to cone tip. | [ ] | [ ] | [ ] |
| 12. Insert cone firmly into stoma toward direction of bowel lumen. Digitally inspect stoma with gloved, lubricated finger before irrigation to determine direction of bowel lumen if necessary. | [ ] | [ ] | [ ] |
| 13. Slowly begin flow of water into stoma, readjust position of cone gently with increasing firmness until there is no leakage around cone. | [ ] | [ ] | [ ] |
| 14. Adjust height of water container to deliver 1000 mL water in 10 to 15 minutes. Bottom of container is even with patient's shoulder if in sitting position. If patient complains of cramps, slow or temporarily stop infusion without removing cone. | [ ] | [ ] | [ ] |
| 15. Clamp tubing and remove cone, closing top of sleeve. Small gush of fluid returns into sleeve followed by intermittent spurts. If return is slow, pour warm water over stoma, massage abdomen, or have patient drink a warm liquid. | [ ] | [ ] | [ ] |
| 16. When majority of feces and water have been evacuated, dry and seal bottom of sleeve. | [ ] | [ ] | [ ] |
| 17. Remove and dispose of gloves, but reglove before beginning following steps. | [ ] | [ ] | [ ] |
| 18. When bowel evacuation has ceased, remove sleeve and set aside for cleansing. | [ ] | [ ] | [ ] |

*(continued)*

© 1992 J.B. Lippincott Company, Fundamentals of Nursing: Human Health and Function

## 38-5: Irrigating A Colostomy *(Continued)*

|  | E | S | U |
|---|---|---|---|
| 19. Clean stoma and skin with warm water. | [ ] | [ ] | [ ] |
| 20. Apply skin barrier and new pouch. | [ ] | [ ] | [ ] |
| 22. Remove and dispose of gloves. Wash hands. | [ ] | [ ] | [ ] |
| 23. Document procedure and observations. | [ ] | [ ] | [ ] |

E = Excels;  S = Satisfactory;  U = Unsatisfactory

COMMENTS:

[ ] Pass  [ ] Fail

Student's Signature_____ Date_____

Instructor's Signature_____ Date _____

© 1992 J.B. Lippincott Company, Fundamentals of Nursing:  Human Health and Function